Mark Christensen

The Seed

Mark Christensen

The Seed

The love story of grandparents raising second generation children

JustFiction Edition

Impressum / Imprint

Bibliografische Information der Deutschen Nationalbibliothek: Die Deutsche Nationalbibliothek verzeichnet diese Publikation in der Deutschen Nationalbibliografie; detaillierte bibliografische Daten sind im Internet über http://dnb.d-nb.de abrufbar.

Alle in diesem Buch genannten Marken und Produktnamen unterliegen warenzeichen-, marken- oder patentrechtlichem Schutz bzw. sind Warenzeichen oder eingetragene Warenzeichen der jeweiligen Inhaber. Die Wiedergabe von Marken, Produktnamen, Gebrauchsnamen, Handelsnamen, Warenbezeichnungen u.s.w. in diesem Werk berechtigt auch ohne besondere Kennzeichnung nicht zu der Annahme, dass solche Namen im Sinne der Warenzeichen- und Markenschutzgesetzgebung als frei zu betrachten wären und daher von jedermann benutzt werden dürften.

Bibliographic information published by the Deutsche Nationalbibliothek: The Deutsche Nationalbibliothek lists this publication in the Deutsche Nationalbibliografie; detailed bibliographic data are available in the Internet at http://dnb.d-nb.de.

Any brand names and product names mentioned in this book are subject to trademark, brand or patent protection and are trademarks or registered trademarks of their respective holders. The use of brand names, product names, common names, trade names, product descriptions etc. even without a particular marking in this works is in no way to be construed to mean that such names may be regarded as unrestricted in respect of trademark and brand protection legislation and could thus be used by anyone.

Coverbild / Cover image: www.ingimage.com

Verlag / Publisher:
JustFiction! Edition
ist ein Imprint der / is a trademark of
AV Akademikerverlag GmbH & Co. KG
Heinrich-Böcking-Str. 6-8, 66121 Saarbrücken, Deutschland / Germany
Email: info@justfiction-edition.com

Herstellung: siehe letzte Seite /
Printed at: see last page
ISBN: 978-3-8454-4956-2

Copyright © 2013 AV Akademikerverlag GmbH & Co. KG
Alle Rechte vorbehalten. / All rights reserved. Saarbrücken 2013

THE SEED

A novel by
Mark A. Christensen

DEDICATION

For you, Elizabeth,

The child all mothers yearn for.

The wife all men would be fortunate to marry.

The mother all children pray for.

The friend all friends should have.

And a grandmother to us all.

You are love's true meaning.

Every June we celebrate Grandparent's Day, but is that enough? One out of every four adults raises a second generation. If it were not for those grandparents and the love they are willing to share, our foster homes and orphanages would be overflowing, our crime rates and the number of children on the street would soar. Can we ever do enough to recognize and celebrate the devotion of these true heroes?

Chapter One

It's the rhythmic hiss and click of the ventilator I remember. I knew the noise was necessary; the machine was pumping oxygen into her, keeping her alive. It should have been a hopeful noise, a signal to me that she still lived, still had a chance, but after days and weeks and months of the constant hiss, click, hiss, it only irritated me.

I could not believe my life would go on without her. Why did the moon continue to shine so brightly? Why did the landscape I saw through her hospital window look unchanged? The world was coming to an end. The woman who had raised me, loved me, and taught me, might leave me.

She has been through so much; her body seemed to be giving up. It's New Year's Day and I had promised to have her home by Christmas. It seems there is no end to the tortures she must endure.

Last night, one of her doctors came in and told me the antibiotics she's been on are causing a massive allergic reaction. This morning I noticed her skin had turned beet red. Her face and arms and hands and legs are swollen so I couldn't even recognize her without the name tag above her bed.

She'd laugh at that, if she were awake. She'd smile and her upper lip would quiver and she'd laugh at the ridiculousness of it all. Liz Ostlund would laugh at the chance to play a great joke on me, her Mark-O. She'd say something like, 'it's pretty neat, Mark-O, my love, I can pretend to be someone else and I don't even need a mask.'

She won't open her eyes today, though. She doesn't seem to know I'm here. "Granny, Granny, my sweetie, it's, Mark," I say over and over again in the hope that she'll respond somehow. <u>Oh, Granny, how did it come to this? I love you so much. How can I let this go on? How can I let them hurt you anymore?</u>

I sit beside her hospital bed and reach through the side rails and under the covers for her swollen hand. I hold it and remember all the wonderful things that hand has done for me through the years. Her warm, maternal touch on my cheek;

her hand resting on my shoulder to ease my pain; that hand holding mine, guiding me through the years.

It was her hands I saw first when I came out of a coma, years ago. Granny told me how it happened, how I got out of bed during the night and got into her pills. She found me, barely breathing and back in my bed.

****

"Mark! Mark! Mark! Please wake up! Mark-o, sweetie, oh god! Liz screamed as she shook the two year old in his crib. He didn't wake. <u>Is he even breathing</u>? She lifted him out of the bed and ran to the living room.

"What's wrong?" George yelped, nearly colliding with them in the hallway.

"It's Mark!" Liz screamed again, "He got into my pills. He won't wake up." She knew time was running out. "Let's go," she ordered.

As she headed toward the door with Mark in her arms, George disappeared down the hall and caught up with her as she reached the car. He was there to open the door and help her get herself and the boy inside, and then he ran to the driver's side.

"Got the empty pill bottles," he said breathlessly as he started the old Ford. She closed her eyes, held Mark tightly in her arms, and prayed repeatedly, "Please let him be okay," as she felt the car lurch backwards out of the drive.

She shook him and talked to him. She begged him to open his eyes, to breathe, to live. She knew they were going very fast. She heard a siren and saw the glare of a red flashing light. George was mumbling something about not stopping for anyone.

She was praying again. "Let him be okay. I beg you, God, let him live."

The louder her prayers were, the faster George seemed to drive. She kept praying. She looked up from Mark's face only briefly as the car careened wildly around a corner and into the hospital entrance drive. She heard the brakes squeal.

George was practically standing on the brake pedal. The car was sliding, the brakes were screeching and George was swearing.

The car stopped, suddenly and within inches of the emergency department door. Liz ran out of the car, still holding the unconscious child in her arms. She was hollering for a doctor before she even got into the hospital.

"Doctor, where's the goddam doctor?"

A nurse came running; her arms open for a hand-off. Liz was too frantic and blinded by fright to understand what to do.

The nurse said firmly, "Ma'am, calm down and give me the child."

Liz hesitated for an instant. She wondered if she would ever hold him again. She handed Mark over and turned to see George behind her.

They followed the nurse into a room that reeked of rubbing alcohol. Kneading the stinging odor and tears from her eyes, Liz looked at the child. He was the still, small center of this roomful of people, equipment and noise. She heard the loudspeaker shout its announcement, "All house doctors, E.R. stat. All doctors, E.R. stat!" That's for him, she thought with a shiver. George must have seen the chill that ran through her. His arms were around her in an instant. She had once thought he had no feelings that his years as a Marine made him immune to pain. Now she felt tears stream down his face as he hugged her close. His tears mingled with hers as they watched the horror before them.

"How many pills did he take?" a nurse shouted over the din as she put a tube down the boys throat. Liz wondered if it would help him breathe. His lips seem so blue.

George was giving the empty pill containers to a nurse.

"I don't know," he said as he shook his head, "I think most of them were filled two weeks ago. Each of them was a thirty day prescription.

The nurse turned towards Mark. Liz backed into a corner of the room with George. She knew she should stay out of the way.

A tall, slender man raced into the room, shouting, "Whaddya got Susan?"

It seemed as if an army of men and women, their stethoscope's dangling from their hands, followed this doctor. Liz heard the tall doctor say, "Let's bag him." She looked away as the nurse hooked a large grey thing to the tube coming out of Mark's throat.   Another man came to her. This man asked them to follow him to a waiting area. Liz said, "No, I'm not leavin' him, not now, not ever." She looked at George and then at Mark. George put his hands on her shoulders and started to talk. Liz didn't want to hear what he had to say. "I'm not leaving him, George," she said emphatically. The man who had asked them to leave tried to talk with her; she put her hands over her ears. She didn't want to hear anymore.

Liz looked at George; tears were running down his face now. His hands were still on her shoulders. He was pleading with her to let the doctors take care of Mark. She could read his lips, he said, "Please Liz, please, honey, let's get out of here for just a little while."

She looked towards Mark for a moment, and then bolted for the door. George was right behind her.

"Give me a damn cigarette," she said as soon as they reached the waiting room.

An aged lady dressed in pink offered some coffee. "Here kids," she said, "looks as if you could use this."

Liz sipped the steaming coffee and took an endlessly long drag on the cigarette George lit for her. Her panic subsided a little as she blew the smoke from her lungs.

She paced and drank black coffee and smoked for the next three hours. Liz went into the hall periodically to watch the door to Mark's room and keep tabs on the comings and goings there. George positioned himself in the doorway of the waiting room, his head turning first in the direction of Mark's room, then towards Liz. Liz watched him through the long, horrible vigil, he never moved from the spot in the door, his head turned either in Mark's direction or hers.

She pictured the different ways all of this could end. Would she ever hold Mark again? Would she be able to give him the love she so desperately wanted to give a child? She knew she would never forgive herself for what had happened. She begged God to save him, promising that Mark would have more love and attention than any child, anywhere, had ever had.

She was sure she had worn the wax from the floor with her continuous pacing. She felt a scream of frustration rising in her,

"Why don't they tell me what's happened to him, George? Why doesn't someone come and tell us how he's doing?" She asked for the hundredth time.

George looked at her and started to say, "I don't..." when three men in green and white hospital clothes entered the waiting room.

"Ostlund's?" One man said aloud.

"That's us," said George quickly.

The men introduced themselves as Doctors Craig, Stephens and Jones. Each of them wore a name pin, Liz noticed. Dr. Stephens had a silver clipboard. He opened it and said,

"Mark took a lot of pills. When he got here he was in respiratory arrest."

"What does that mean?" Liz asked.

"That means he wasn't breathing." Dr. Jones answered.

"Oh my God! No." Liz screamed, turning as white as the doctor's coats.

"Shhhh," said George soothingly, as he rubbed the palm of her hand. "Shhh."

Everyone was silent for a moment. Liz took a deep breath and realized what they told her was serious, but, she thought with a glimmer of hope forming, they haven't said that he's dead.

"Is he dead?" She asked outright, wanting to know one way or another, right now.

"No," said Stephens, "We pumped his stomach and had to hook him up to a respirator. He's holding his own, now."

Liz just stood there. She stared at Stephens until she could force the words from her throat, "Is my Mark-O going to make it?"

The doctor answered, "Ma' am, we're doing all we can for him right now, but, Mark is only breathing eight times a minute. The normal is twenty-five to thirty for a child his age."

Dr. Jones added, "I'm not going to sit here and give you much hope, which would be foolish of me. If I were you, I would admit that the situation is serious."

He continued, "To be honest...If I was in your position, I'd be making funeral arrangements. I don't see much hope for recovery. He took too many pills and they stayed in his system way too long."

"No, no, no," Liz cried uncontrollably. "He'll come through. I know him. He'll come through. You'll see. I'm not making any funeral arrangements. No, sir. You'll see." She took only one sharp breath in, then pointed her finger at the three and said, "I'll see my Mark-o back to health. He'll walk out of here holdin' my hand. He loves me and I love him that little heart of his is full of love and love'll keep it beatin'. You'll see."

Dr. Jones answered, "That's fine, I hope that happens, but it is our job to tell you what we expect, what is medically realistic."

Liz nodded a quiet affirmation. She understood perfectly, it was the doctors who didn't understand.

"Where's Mark at?" George asked.

"He's in ICU," answered Dr. Stephens. "The nurse will direct you." He said while pointing to a nurse as she entered the waiting room.

Doctors Jones and Craig turned to leave the Ostlund's. Dr. Stephens put a warm hand on Liz' shoulder and said, "Please, know how truly sorry we are. You can rest assured, even though things look bleak; we're still going to do all we can for Mark."

"Appreciate it Doctor," said George as he extended his hand to Stephens, first, then the other two. He thanked them all.

Liz sighed deeply as the doctors left. The room was very quiet. Part of her wanted to rush to Mark's side, part of her was afraid of seeing him so ill. She turned her eyes upward and said in a whisper, "Please don't take him from us. We need him, God, and he needs us. Let me, me and George bring him back to health. Please God."

George waited quietly until she had finished her prayer, then he held out his hand to her. "It's time. Let's go be with him, honey," he said.

They walked down the long hallway, hand in hand. ICU was at the end of the hallway, the source of glaring lights and loud noises. Liz dreaded each step, at the beginning of that walk. <u>Mark-o would look different. Would he be all right? How would she bare to watch him suffer so,</u> she thought, but as they got closer she realized her Mark would need her, would only get well if she were there and in those thoughts she found her strength. <u>Mark needs me. I'll be there to get him well.</u>

She held George's hand tightly as they entered the ICU room.

Liz gasped quickly as she got her first glimpse of her boy. It looked as if a plumbing store had exploded around his tiny body. Tubing and hoses crisscrossed the crib. She noticed a constant hiss, click, hiss that seemed to come from the machine at Mark's bedside. She figured it was the 'respirator,' the doctors had spoken of.

A woman's voice seemed to come from nowhere. Liz felt a hand on her shoulder, she turned to see a woman in green ask,

"Are you the Ostlund's?"

"Yes, yes, I'm George, she's Liz, and this is our boy, Mark." George stammered.

"I'm the charge nurse in ICU, Anne Bristow," she said and paused briefly, "we have Mark's hands tied to the bed, so if he wakes he won't pull any of the tubes out."

Liz felt a breath of hope rush through her. <u>They must be expecting him to wake up, not die, if they tied his hands down.</u> Liz smiled at George and he smiled back. She figured he had the same thought. They had been together for so many years, she knew they often thought the same way; finished one another's sentences, too.

Liz watched and listened as the nurse explained some of the tubing and paraphernalia around Mark. <u>She cares about him, I can tell,</u> she thought. It was another small burden lifted from Liz's shoulders.

The nurse left the room eventually with the promise, "someone will be in every fifteen minutes to check on Mark and that all of his vital signs are being constantly monitored at the center of the unit."

Liz felt abandoned when she left. It was as if hope had left the room with her. She had to face the horrible fact that Mark was barely alive. She watched his tiny chest move up and down in time to the hiss, click of the big machine. She looked at the lines of fluid going in and out of his small body and wondered how he would ever come back to her.

"Liz, honey," said George, suddenly, out of the white noise of machinery, "Liz, let's pray."

She looked at her husband and smiled her warmest smile. He always seemed to know what to do to make her feel better. He always knew what to say.

She knelt right down next to Mark's bed, putting her arm through the side rails and gathering his chubby fist in hers.

They prayed and she knew Mark had to have heard their prayers, even if he was close to heaven. She hoped her pleas might pull him right back to where he belonged, with her.

She sat beside him, after the prayers. She still held Mark's hand in hers. George pulled another chair to the bedside and sat next to her. They sat without saying a word. For hours, they sat watching Mark and his machines. The nurses came and went. The hands on the clock on the wall moved so slowly Liz imagined time had truly stopped when Mark stopped breathing. She knew this was only the beginning of a long and difficult wait.

"Liz, honey," George said gently at three a.m., "Liz, we should go home, get a little sleep. We don't know how long he'll need us to be here for him. We gotta keep up our strength. Ya know, we're not kids anymore. We gotta take care of ourselves for Mark."

She was horrified when he first said it. She wanted to shout a loud, "No," at the thought of leaving Mark-o alone. What if something went wrong? Or, what if he woke-up and needed us. He'd never forgive me if I wasn't here when he needed me." Those were her first thoughts. Then she looked at her husband. He looked terrible. His face looked grey in the strange light from the monitor.

Maybe, maybe I should get him home, she thought, worried about the toll such a night was taking on George. He loved Mark, too. She knew that for sure. She looked at her watch to confirm the late hour.

"George, how are you feeling?" She asked, "I'm afraid to leave him alone, but maybe you're right about saving our strength.

She had to admit to herself, even if she didn't say it to George, the night and all of it's tragedy had worn her out, too. Still...

George put his arm around her and whispered, "I know he'll be all right for the rest of tonight. I just know it. You need some rest, honey. Let's go home."

She hesitated only a moment longer; then, she rose from the chair and bent over Mark's bed.

"Love, I'll be back in the morning. You hang in there, kid-o, you promise me, now. You're going to get better real soon."

She patted his hand and pulled the sheet over his arms. She placed her pink lips gently on his cool, rounded cheek to kiss him good-bye.

Liz stood straight after kissing the boy and started moving backward, slowly. She didn't want to take her eyes off the little face she loved so dearly. She could feel the tears running down her own face, but she never made a sound.

They got home and crawled into the bed they shared without speaking. Liz knew there was nothing to say. She knew George was aching for their boy just as she was.

She never slept that night. She lay awake watching the dim light from the street play across the ceiling of their room. Thoughts of how life would be without Mark kept threatening to break, fully formed into consciousness. She would not let them.

She began a silent litany. Mouthing the words so as not to wake her husband.

"My kiss was magic, Mark," she said silently, in the darkness. "I'll bring you home. I'll bring you home. I promise you, I'll bring you home," she said over and over again. If there was any magic left in the world, Liz was sure she could make it answer her command.

At six she crawled out of bed. The phone hadn't rung through the night. She felt that was both a bad, and a good sign. It meant Mark had not gotten worse. It also meant he had not wakened from his coma.

They were at the hospital, she and George, by seven. She took her place at Mark's bedside and once again poked her hand through the side rails to grasp his fist.

It was the beginning of the unchanging pattern of their days.

A week went by and Mark continued to sleep. Liz noticed his lips were no longer blue and his hand seemed somehow stronger in hers, but he did not wake. The doctors were less and less optimistic as the days went on. They would tell her the longer Mark slept the less chance he would ever wake. She refused to listen to such nonsense and told several of the medical men just that. She and George continued their vigil.

On Wednesday, ten days after Mark's accident, Doctor Jones once again gave a dire prediction.

"Mrs. Ostlund I don't know, but each day he sleeps his chances are less. If he does ever wake up, he may have extensive brain damage. All we can do now is pray."

Liz took that as a challenge. As soon as the doctor left she was down on her knees at Mark's bedside. She lowered the side rail, first, so that she could pull his hand to her. Don't know what the stupid side rails are for anyway, they think he won't go anywhere. He's in a coma, for God's sake.

George knelt beside her. She had Mark's hands between hers and between her prayers she'd open her hands and kiss his tiny one. She thought how much life he would miss if he never awakened. She had plans for his life, days to spend just enjoying him and a wonderful life to share with him. He had to wake up, he just had to. She decided to keep praying, right there on her knees, she'd keep praying and probably crying until Mark woke up.

****

I still remember the moment so clearly! Granny and George were kneeling beside my bed that day. I turned my head a little, I heard their voices and I saw her hands folded in prayer at my side. I looked to their faces and saw their eyes were closed, tears were running down Granny's face, both of their voices were soft with pleading for my recovery.

I looked at Granny's hands again and asked her if we were still going to the park. No one heard me. Granny was holding one of my hands and I pulled it away from her and said, "Are we going to the park now."

Granny and George opened their eyes suddenly, then. They just stayed where they were and looked at me as if I rose from the dead. I really surprised them!

It was their prayers that pulled me through. I hope my prayers can save her now.

****

After the pill-taking incident, Granny told me things went pretty smoothly. I was still staying with her and George; my own parents were so young. They didn't feel ready to take on raising me. My dad is Granny and George's son, Albert, he and my mother, Nacole, were married when they were sixteen, I came along in the first nine months they were married. They just weren't ready for me, Granny always said.

So, Granny and George agreed to keep me and raise me as their own for as long as Albert and Nacole allowed it. Albert joined the Air Force and would be stationed in Germany for years. It worked out fine with me. I loved Granny and George as much as, or more, than any kid had ever loved any parent. I had never known any different. When I was really little, I thought they were my mom and dad. I still think of them that way.

****

It was a beautiful, clear, cool Montana morning. Liz stuck her head out the window of the old station wagon, just to feel the crisp air rush past. It was late spring and Liz knew it would warm up as soon as the morning was past. Now was the time to soak up the pine scented air and mountain scenery.

George was taking them to a little town he had worked in years ago after a stint in the Marines and a trip to China. "Look, Mark," George said as he pointed to a two-story, paint faded structure on a side street of Livingston, "that's where I worked as a cook."

Liz felt a glow of warmth and contentment start in her chest and spread through her body whenever she watched her husband tell his stories to the boy. She put both hands to her cheeks to check if they were as hot as they felt from the inside. George looked at her as she did that and smiled, he grabbed one of her hands and kissed the palm. He knew how she felt.

Mark seemed to be listening intently in the back seat. His face and hands rested on the back of the front seat, right in the middle, between his grandparents.

"Here's where I cooked my first Thanksgiving turkey," George said proudly as he pointed to a place with a sign that said, 'Mary's Cafe.'

Liz noticed Mark oohing and ahing appropriately whenever George expounded on his ties with the town. It was so different with their own three children. They took

Saturday trips, then, too, but Lisa, Lee Ann, and Albert spent the time fighting amongst themselves or complaining bitterly about being confined for the long, 'boring' trip.

Not Mark, thought Liz as she looked at the eight year old face hanging over the back of the car seat. Liz wondered how many times they had been forced to call off adventures because her own kids were so obnoxious. The thought of their constant unhappiness and disrespect for George brought fresh pain to Liz. How had she and George failed so miserably at raising their own three children when they seemed, at least, so far, to be so successful at raising Mark?

She noticed they were turning off the main highway, onto a dirt road. Liz was chewing gum, a frequent pleasure.

George always told her he could tell when she was getting angry or anxious or upset. "That gum of yours snaps and pops whenever you're workin' up a temper. Your jaws move so fast it's a wonder the gum stays in there and doesn't get shot across the room with all the force you put into it."

George looked at her, now, and put his hand on her knee. "Relax will ya honey. I just wanna show Mark where I sold my cosmetics."

Liz had to chuckle at George's perception. I must be chewing even harder than usual. He knows I don't like to come to this part of town. Why does he insist on doing this? Oh, well, she thought as she went back to chewing vigorously, snapping and popping her gum as much as possible. Huh! That'll show him, she thought and stammered, "And if you don't quit playing with my leg... I'll....I'll... I'll... well you think you've heard me snap my gum, before, that wasn't nothing. I'll never give you any peace. "What cosmetics?" Mark begged.

George pointed towards the ramshackle houses on this gravel road they were traveling on.

"When my apartment rent came due every month, I'd grab my bag of cosmetics and walk in all these cat houses," George said with a smile draped on his face. "Jesus, I could make the money down here," he finished.

Mark started laughing as soon as George finished. Liz wasn't sure he knew what 'cat houses' were and Liz didn't think he needed to know.

"Oh my God, George. Get the H out of this red light district before you corrupt the child for good."

Mark's head turned to his grandfather and he said, "What's a red light district?"

"Honey," Liz growled, "you're gonna have to wait till you're a little older before I tell you that. Your Granddad doesn't always use his head."

"That's what you always say, 'when you're older I'll tell you.' When will I ever be older enough?" Mark asked in a very serious eight year old voice. "I'm gonna have so much to learn, 'when I'm older,' I won't have any time to do anything else!" he said with obvious consternation.

Liz looked at the cherubic little face of her solemn grandson and burst out laughing. She felt like the luckiest woman in the world. She put her hands on either side of Mark's face, squeezing his adorable cheeks just a bit, then she planted a big, juicy kiss right on his red lips. No doubt about it, she was blest. Liz learned over the years to enjoy her grandson and the happiness he brought to her home. There were times when she could almost forget the pain her own three children had caused her. George told her he loved every moment of seeing her smiling and laughing and playing with Mark.

She was always anxious for snow season to begin. <u>The winters don't seem so hard at all when I have Mark to share them with.</u>

Liz stood at the living room windows. She was watching for Mark to walk from the bus stop, but she was also enjoying the view. George had built this home for her and she often lingered at the picture window that faced the front lawn.

It was her favorite room, filled with her parents' antiques and facing the huge corner lot ringed with tall pines. In the summer the scent from the trees filled the rooms of the house and in the winter their dark green boughs broke the wind and kept a little of the blowing snow from the Ostlund drive and walkways.

She caught a glimpse of the dark yellow school bus as it whizzed past the pines and came to a screeching halt a few houses away. Mark would be running down the drive any minute.

Liz usually made a point of picking Mark up from school, but today she had planned a surprise and as soon as the bus passed she put on her coat, hat, scarf and mittens and rushed out the door.

She gathered up a huge handful of the freshly fallen winter white and hid behind the tree nearest the entrance to the drive.

She waited there, listening to children's voices as they passed.

Soon, she heard the familiar footfall of her own grandson and as he turned into the drive she met him with a playfully thrown snowball to the chest.

"Hey, what the...," Mark said as the snow hit him. "Granny, is that you?" he said as he smiled one of his best smiles when he saw her.

"Gottcha," Liz said as she bent to scoop up more snow. "You better run my little Mark-o, Granny's gonna get you!" She said as she pitched another soft snowball at the defenseless and laughing boy.

She followed the surprise romp in the snow with hot cocoa and a freshly baked apple pie. She knew how much Mark loved her pies, baking them and watching him eat was pure pleasure. It was afternoons like this that almost made up for the sad years she had spent raising her own children.

Liz worked part-time at the local Sears store. She tried to work while Mark was in school, but whenever she worked evenings she knew George and Mark had their own special time. She loved walking into the house and finding Mark on George's lap in the old recliner in front of the fire. They'd either be sound asleep, one trying to out-snore the other, or they'd be gabbing. George could tell endless stories, about his time in the Marines, or about their own kids and what it was like raising them. Mark asked a million questions, seemed like he was always asking questions.

<u>I wonder how I'll find them tonight,</u> Liz thought as she drove home on the snow covered roads. The store had been extra busy and she stayed to help close up. She pulled in the Ostlund driveway just after eleven. <u>I love the snow, but I hate retail this time of year,</u> she thought as she parked the car and started towards the house, <u>November, Christmas shoppers, yuck.</u>

She was in a definitely grumpy mood as she opened the front door and started to stomp the snow off her boots.

"Hey, Granny, we missed you!"

She heard Mark say those words, Liz looked into the living room and felt her grouchiness melt away. Her guys were in their chair with the firelight washing them in gold and orange.

"Well, you two make quite a pretty picture;" Liz answered as she took off her boots and hung her coat in the front closet.

She walked into the living room, gave a strong hug to Mark and a big kiss to her husband and perched on the arm of the recliner. "You two are sure wide awake this evening. What'ya been up to?"

"George has been telling me 'bout the day I was born. Were you really happy, Granny?"

"Happy, happy? We were lots more than just happy, weren't we George?"

"Like I tol' ya, Mark, I've never seen your Granny chew her gum so hard in her life. Why, just before the doctor came out to tell us you were here, Granny was chewin' and poppin' and grumblin' about it takin' too long and why weren't the doctors doin' something. I was sure that big ol' wad of gum was gonna fly outta her mouth any second." George said as he looked at Liz and smiled.

"Now, George, don't exaggerate so."

"Exaggerate, I never exaggerate. Besides, that's not the best part of the story. I already tol' Mark the best part. Tell Granny what I told you."

Liz looked at George, who had an enormous grin on his face, and knew he had probably told Mark quite a tale.

"Go ahead Mark-o, tell me what George's been tellin' you.

"Well," Mark started, "George said when the doctor finally came out to tell you I was born and I was a beautiful boy baby," (Liz watched Mark's adorable face as he emphasized the 'beautiful boy baby' part), "Well, Granny, George says you sucked in a big breath, you were so happy and surprised, and when you sucked in that breath, you sucked in that big lump of gum, too, and the doctor had to do somethin' called the Hemlock on you to get that gum out so you wouldn't die. But, George said he was laughin' the whole time 'cuz he warned you all day 'bout chewin' that gum so much and gettin' so excited. He said he couldn't help you at all, cuz it was just what he said would happen."

Liz realized she had gum in her mouth now; she self-consciously stopped chewing and looked at Mark, then at George. She wanted George to think she was still a little mad for him laughing at her that way, why, she could have choked to death.

"Oh, you two!" She said finally, watching as the two in the chair seemed to breathe a sigh of relief. "George you do exaggerate, at least, a little," she said as she started to giggle at the memory of the day and at Mark's story telling. She reached out to Mark and tickled his tummy just once, and then she kissed the top of his head. All three of them laughed together for awhile. <u>It was good to be home, good to have such a wonderful family,</u> Liz thought.

Chapter Two

"Granny, Granny, come on sweetie, you've just gotta wake up. I know you're tired, but you just gotta keep trying."

I keep talking to her; keep trying to tell her to get well, to fight. I don't know if it does any good, but I think she knows, at least, that I'm here.

She was always there for me, every time I needed her, I didn't even have to ask, she just knew the right things to say. Now, I don't know what the 'right thing to say' is.

The doctors told us today that she's allergic to every antibiotic they try. She's got some kind of infection and every time they try a new drug on her, her body just can't take it. The doctor today told me he called in another specialist to see if they can't beat this thing. They've only got one more antibiotic to try. I keep prayin' and pleadin', but I just don't know anymore.

****

<u>It's been a cold winter, so far,</u> Liz thought as she dried the dishes and waited for Mark to come home from school. This was her favorite time of day, seeing him burst in the door, listening to every detail of his day, watching him devour whatever special treat she made.

She thought back to when her two oldest children were Mark's age. Albert and Lisa never seemed happy to be home from school. When she was still married to their father, she could certainly understand. That drunken bum always had the house in turmoil, but once she met and married George, why did the kids continue to want to pull away. George lavished as much love on them as he did on their own daughter, Lee Ann, and as much as he did on Mark, now.

What was the difference? She and George hadn't changed; they had lived for the kids. They wanted nothing more than to share their love and a family life with all of them. Albert and Lisa wanted nothing to do with any of that and were gone as soon as they were sixteen. Lee Ann married and left as soon as she could, too. <u>I wonder what we did so different for them,</u> Liz continued to ponder as she waited for Mark. <u>I had so much love to give them and it seemed like they just kept throwing it back in my face. Thank God for Mark, I know he loves us,</u> she thought as her grandson walked through the door shouting, "Anybody home? I'm home Granny!"

She rushed to the living room to greet him.

"Granny, I gotta talk to you and George, today, okay?"

"Sure, sweetie, have you got a problem?"

"Well, sort of, I mean, I got questions and the teacher said stuff I don't understand."

Liz was concerned; Mark had heard things before from people at school, things that bothered him. He had always come to her and George, though. They had always been able to help him sort things out.

"George is in the basement, why don't you go get him and we can all talk over a piece of peach pie."

Mark smiled broadly, kissed his grandmother, and ran for the basement stairs. She knew he'd be fine; he was such a happy kid that whatever the problem was, she was sure they would solve it. It took several mouthfuls of the feathery crust and warm, sweet peaches before Mark started his story. Liz watched his face as he described what his teacher, Mrs. Allen, had said that afternoon.

"Gramps," he began slowly, "Gramps, Mrs. Allen asked me why you and Grandma haven't adopted me."

Liz noticed Mark had stopped chewing but never took his eyes off his plate.

"I didn't know why. She seemed kinda nosy about it or somethin'. She told me that usually a kid gets 'dopted if he lives with somebody as long as I've lived with you." He paused and then looked up at his grandfather, "Gramps, I don't know why you never 'dopted me and that's what I tol' creepy ol' Mrs. Allen. But...well, could you tell me why?"

George motioned to Mark who had put down his fork and seemed on the verge of tears. Mark got out of his chair and went around the table to his grandfather. George pulled the boy up onto his lap.

Liz continued to look on. As she listened to her husband the old familiar flush of love washed over her. George was a wonderful man and he continued to prove it, time and time again.

"Mark," George said as he cupped the boys chin in his big hand, "I want to tell you what I believe about adoption. It's what Granny believes, too, but I guess I have more personal experience with this particular thing," he said as he turned Mark just a bit in his lap so he could hold him within the circle of his arms.

"Mark, usually it's people who can't have children of their own who adopt. They adopt children whose parents couldn't take care of them or maybe the parents have died and the children need a new home with parents to love them. That part is kinda like us. I mean, Albert and Nacole couldn't take care of you in the best way and they knew that, so they asked us to act as your parents, to give you lots of love. That make sense to ya?"

Mark nodded silently.

George looked at Liz and smiled, then he continued, "My brother and me, we were a little like you to. I mean, our mother couldn't take care of us. We were born when times were really hard. She knew she wouldn't be able to feed us or get us the clothes we needed, so she wanted us to be adopted by someone who could."

"Did you get adopted Gramps?" asked Mark.

"Well, we did, but we weren't as lucky as you. We went to a big place called an orphanage for awhile. They took good care of us there but there were so many kids, well, we got enough food and warm clothes, but not much love."

Mark never took his eyes off his grandfather's face.

"I can remember crying each night before we went to sleep, hoping for a home where we'd have real parents."

"Then what happened, Gramps?"

"Well, eventually we did get adopted, but me and my brother had to be separated. He had to go to a different home and be adopted by different parents."

"Geez," said Mark quietly.

"Mark, I've spent my life wondering where my brother is, what he looks like, what kind of man he's become, and the sad thing is that a lot of kids whose own parents can't care for them are going through the same thing my brother and I did."

"What'd'ya mean, Gramps?"

"Well, take our kids; did you know Albert and Lisa aren't my own kids?"

"No, did'ya 'dopt um?" Mark asked.

"Well, I did. See, Liz, your granny, was married before and she had Lisa and Albert when she was married to that other man. He wasn't any good, though. He drank all the time and wouldn't work and eventually left Granny and Lisa and Albert. He didn't want his family, I guess."

"So you saved'um, right!" said Mark.

"Well, I guess you could say that. I just kept remembering me and my brother and when I first met Liz I knew how hard it was for her to take care of those kids. She had to work at the store all the time and try to make enough money to feed'em and buy clothes and all. She used just break down and cry when we first met. I think she was all tired out from trying so hard."

George looked over at Liz again, she felt their eyes connect. <u>You did save me and the kids, George, I would'a had to give them up for adoption if you hadn't come along.</u>

23

George looked back at the little boy in his lap and smiled.

"I kept thinking how she might have to give those kids up for adoption if she stayed alone, and how those kids might be put in different homes someday. I couldn't let that happen, besides I loved her right from the start. So I married your granny and adopted Albert and Lisa, now they are my own kids."

"So...why don't you 'dopt me, then Gramps, since you're kinda used to doin' it." Mark said quickly.

Liz had to hold back a chuckle on that one, she noticed George trying not to laugh too.

"Good question, big guy. Remember though, you still have two good parents who will be able to take care of you someday. I'd adopt you in a minute if you didn't. I think it's so sad when kids have to get stuck in foster homes or institutions, when no one wants them or doesn't want brothers and sisters together. Where are their grandparents? Why can't the grandparents take them in? Can you imagine how many orphanages and foster homes would close if the kids own grandparents would adopt them. Yup, it's just too bad more people in this country don't think about those poor kids."

"Yeah, too bad more kids don't have a Granny and a George like you guys." Mark said brightly.

"But you, young man have parents who just needed a little more time to learn to be grown up and until they're ready, we're here for ya, but we'd never want to take you away from lovin' Albert and Nacole. We'll just love ya lots 'til they can make a family for you. That's why we don't adopt ya. Sound okay, Mark?"

"Sounds great, Gramps, I get you guys to love me annnnnnnd Albert and Nacole too. Hey, it's like havin' four parents. Not many kids have that, do they?"

"No they don't son, you're very lucky." Liz chimed in.

"If your teacher doesn't understand, you tell her to call me, personal, ya hear?"

George said, then summed it all up with a happy, "hey, that ball game is on this afternoon, ya up for a little sports watchin'?"

"You're on, Gramps," said Mark.

Liz got out of her chair just ahead of George and gave him a big kiss on the cheek. She had never been so happy.

"Granny how come your mouth looks funny?" Mark asked.

Liz straightened up after kissing George, her vision clouded with tears of happiness.

"What'd'ya mean Mark-o?" She said.

"Oh, that's just Granny for ya," George chimed in right away. "Whenever she's so happy she can't hold it, she either cries or her upper lip quivers like that. You watch Mark, you can always tell when she's gettin' sentimental," he said as he looked at Liz and smiled.

"That's about enough of both of you, now go watch your game," Liz said as she quickly wiped an errant tear from her cheek. George was right, of course, but she certainly didn't want to admit it to Mark. No need for him to have her all figured out. "You two are just gettin' too smart for your own britches!" She said as she finally shooed them out of her kitchen.

****

"Mark, I'm Dr. Beck," he said as if he were greeting me at a cocktail party. This guy who just operated on her for the third time. He just seemed a little too casual, at first. I guess I shouldn't have been so quick to judge.

"Your grandmother has been through a lot, I know, but I think she'll turn the corner with this surgery. Part of her lung had become just a source of constant infection; no antibiotic could've cleaned it up. We got rid of all the dead tissue and the good thing was that we saw no more signs of cancer. I think with that infected tissue gone, she has a much better chance. She seems like a real fighter. She makes me want to fight hard for her."

I thanked him for the news and then settled in to wait for Granny to come back from the recovery room. I knew not to expect any real change right away, but I gotta admit it was hard to see her wheeled in the same ICU room with the ventilator still pumping away. I had hoped she'd be even the very tiniest bit more responsive, but as I squeezed her cool hand, I knew the wait would continue.

****

It was Valentine's Day. Liz had spent the day cooking a very special dinner for her men. George loved a nice pot roast. The browned potatoes and carrots she cooked with the roast were also his favorites. She pictured him sitting down to tonight's dinner and devouring it. He'd always finish and then push away from the table while patting his stomach and say, "Liz, you can sure cook. This is my favorite kind of meal."

As she checked today's roast, she realized everything she cooked seemed to be his favorite.

She finished trimming the crust to tonight's apple pie when she heard the school bus going past. <u>Mark will be in the house in seconds.</u>

She looked with satisfaction on the dining room table, the red napkins and candles certainly made it look special. She figured Mark would enjoy the small package of heart-shaped candy she had left at his place. She considered that Mark and George might think she was being silly. Were the candles, little presents, pretty napkins, too much? <u>They might laugh a little or tease me, but I have a feeling they both like the attention. Anyways, I like doing this for my sweeties.</u>

"Granny," she heard Mark's voice from the front hall, "Granny, where are you, I'm home.

"In here, Mark, I'm in here, angel," Liz said as she went to meet him.

"Happy Valentine's Day, Granny!" Mark said as he presented her with a small potted violet. He seemed so proud of his gift and she was overwhelmed with the beauty of the little plant.

"Just what I need to chase away the winter chill. It's beautiful Mark. Did you grow it at school?"

"Yup, we all grew one to give to our moms. I love you, Granny."

Liz's heart felt like it did a double flip. She tried hard to keep her upper lip from quivering but she knew that might be impossible.

"Mark-o, you are the sweetest, ever," she said as she bent over to plant a kiss on Mark's baby-like cheeks.

"I've got a little surprise for you, too," she said as she led him out to the table, to show him the special setting and then into the kitchen for a peek in the oven.

"Is that apple pie, Granny?" He asked as he looked at the bubbling dessert.

"Sure is. What else would I make for my special boy on this special day?" she asked.

Mark hugged her ferociously as soon as the oven door was closed. Liz loved these hugs and every time he did it she wondered how long she'd have them, or him. He was eight and a half now. Sometimes when she and George talked about things, George would remind her that Albert and Nacole might ask for Mark any time. How could she bear to let him go after eight and a half years and so many wonderful hugs?

George came in the door a few minutes after Mark.

"And where have you been?" Liz asked playfully as the big man made his way into the kitchen.

"Well, I had a feeling there was somethin' important about today. I left on a very important errand and ended up bringing this home."

With an ear-to-ear grin on his face, George held out a small, square wrapped package.

"Oh, now, what have you gone and done, George? What is all this?" Liz said, feeling a little flustered with all the attention.

"Oh, do you mean you don't want anything? I'm sorry, I thought today was Valentine's Day, but if you aren't interested, well, that's okay," George said, still grinning.

"Now you just stop that!" Liz quipped.

George kept the little package in his right hand and raised his hand above his head. Liz swiped at it a couple of times, but all five feet four inches of her could never reach past George's six feet two inch frame.

"George, you let me have that now! That's enough playing around."

"Oh, so now you're interested. Well keep trying." George said with no move to lower his arm.

Liz had almost had enough playing, "George Ostlund, you lower your arm this instant or I'll never cook another pot roast or make another apple pie as long as I live."

George lowered his arm and presented his gift.

Liz took the small package and opened it slowly. It was a ring. A beautiful sapphire ring. George knew she admired this very ring at the jewelry store in the mall. She had never told him how much she loved it. She had only shown it to him once, when they were Christmas shopping. He had remembered!

<u>Damn! I bet my lip is really doin' a dance.</u> She thought as she stood, ring in hand.

"Well, put it on, honey." George said.

"Yeah, Granny, put it on. We wanna see ya wear it," Mark added.

Liz felt as if her breath had been sucked right out of her.

"Gramps, look at her lip, it's really goin' now." Mark said with a chuckle.

George knew how she felt, how touched she was, he must have because he took her arm and led her to the sofa. Then, he took the ring from her hand and placed it on her finger.

"Looks like it always belonged right there," he said very softly.

Liz kissed him long and hard and then reached for Mark and gave him a big kiss right on his forehead.

"Oh, yuck, this is getting too mushy for me! Yuck, germs! Granny, I'm gettin' too old for you to kiss me and you're too old to be kissin' George like that!"

Mark's remarks started George laughing.

"Son, one day you'll want every pretty lady you see to be kissin' you like that," George giggled.

"Not me, no way, not ever," was Mark's emphatic reply.

****

It was the coldest winter I can remember, now it's the hottest May we've ever had. Montana's never been this hot, even in August, Liz thought as she watched Mark come down the walk, towards home.

"I gotta swim, it's the only way to cool down after a long day of work," he said as he squeezed past her and headed directly to the basement steps.

"That's some greeting, Mark-o," she said to tease him, "I don't rate a kiss anymore, I suppose?"

She heard no response and figured he was already in his basement bedroom, changing for a swim. He was something. She thought it was funny, how he had said, "it's the only way to cool down after a long day of work." I suppose to a eight year old, school is work. He sounds just like George, that's probably where he got it.

"Last one in's a rotten egg," said Mark as he rushed up the stairs, planted a kiss on Liz's cheek and ran out the back door towards the pool.

Liz liked the spring, even a hot one like this. She liked winter, too, but spring and the flowers it seemed especially nice. She loved to watch Mark splash around in the pool. "Look at me, Granny," he would say over and over again as he practiced new ways to play and swim in the tepid water.

Each warm day, Mark's rapid entrance and dip in the pool became the routine. Liz spent every minute she could, watching him from a lawn chair in the backyard. The sun warmed her shoulders as she watched her beloved Mark-o, 'cool off after a long day at work.'

May also brought Mother's Day and Mark always made that day really special for Liz.

"Keep your eyes closed, Granny," he said on the Friday before Mother's Day during that unusually hot spring. "Keep walkin', I'll make sure you don't run into anything," he said.

"Be careful, Mark, ya know I'm not as young as I used to be and I don't want to fall and break a hip or anything."

She heard Mark laugh lightly as she continued to let him lead her, only peeking occasionally, just to make sure he wasn't leading her into a wall or something.

"Okay, now open your eyes real slow," he said.

Liz opened her eyes and found herself standing in front of the living room coffee table.

<u>Oh, it's too beautiful,</u> she thought as she put her hand to her mouth in utter surprise.

"Mark, this is the most wonderful gift I've ever gotten! Oh, sweetie," she said as she quickly bent over to give him a hug.

"Oh, no," Mark said, before Liz could reach his face, "I forgot about the kisses!"

And kiss him she did. She kept kissing him and crying and telling him how much she loved it. She asked him how he ever made such a wonderful Mother's Day basket. "How did you know yellow roses were my absolute, best ever, without-a-doubt favorite," she said between kisses.

"Okay, okay, I guess I know you like it. Enough kisses, okay?" Mark said with a smile.

"Oh, Mark, this is so beautiful." Liz said again as she sat on the couch to continue admiring his gift.

"Granny, your lip's quivering, please don't cry, you know I can't stand to see you cry," he said as he sat down beside her.

"Oh, you're right, no reason for tears. I love you Mark. No mother on earth could ever have a better son. Do you know that?"

"Now I do," said Mark with his best impish grin.

Liz looked at his face. His cheeks were still baby-round, his dimples punctuated the corners of his smile, and his green eyes lit up the room. She would never forget this moment, or the joy he brought her every day.

"I did just happen to make an apple pie today. Something told me we'd want to celebrate. How 'bout a big piece, right now?"

"Yeah!" he said enthusiastically as they both got up from the sofa and headed to the kitchen.

Mark did not need any prompting in order to clean his plate. Liz watched him eat the first few mouthfuls. He was a slow, careful eater and he never paused to take a breath. His mouth was continually full.

She sat and watched him and loved him as she sat with him.

Her heart felt almost unbearably full. She thought of the sunny yellow roses he had filled the basket with. Yellow roses seemed to mark quite a few of the passages of her life. She had carried a small bouquet of them when she and George married. Her father gave her a corsage of yellow roses on her high-school graduation day and she had put yellow roses on his grave.

She could almost see that day again. She was twenty-eight and her father had died so suddenly. She had told him she was pregnant with his grandchild just a week before he was gone. She loved her father so much and now she'd never see him again. She remembered what she prayed as she knelt beside his casket, at the grave site.

"Daddy, here's your favorite flower, a yellow rose. It's a nice big one. I hope you're still able, somehow, to smell it's sweet fragrance. I hope you've found peace. I love you, Daddy.

<u>Oh, lord, am I cryin' again,</u> Liz thought as she quickly wiped her cheek. Mark was finishing the last of his pie and it seemed he hadn't noticed her tears. They were really tears of happiness, she was sure. It was just that yellow roses always made her sentimental. They had been, after all, the one flower her father always grew in his garden.

"Granny, you look sad. What's wrong, don't you like the May basket?" Mark asked as he scraped the last bits of pastry from his plate.

"Sad, no I'm not sad. I was remembering my daddy. He always grew yellow roses and your basket reminded me of him."

"Do you miss him?" Mark asked.

"Oh, boy do I ever miss him, Mark-o. I don't think you ever get over missin' someone you love that's died."

"Granny, you're not goin' die are ya? I mean, are you and George gonna be alive 'til I grow up. I don't wanna ever be away from you and George.

"Oh, Mark-o, of course we will be here. We're not that old, ya know." Liz answered.

"But, Granny, I got a question. How cum you never see your own kids, I mean, I know Albert is in Germany, but what about Lisa and Lee Ann? They never see you or send you Mother's Day presents or anything."

This was going to be hard, Liz knew. How could she explain something she, herself, could not understand.

"Mark, I don't know what to tell you. I've tried for years to figure out why my own children have turned out the way they have. George and I taught them the same things we teach you, about being respectful and loving towards your family. We loved Albert and Lisa and Lee Ann just like we love you. Yet, all three of them have kinda turned their backs on us. Even when they lived at home, they wouldn't do what we asked or be much a part of our family life. I don't know why."

"But, Granny, I don't know why they would do that. You and George are so good to me and us three love each other so much," Mark said with a question in his voice.

"Honey, if I had an answer for that I'd maybe be able to put this family back together, once and for all. But, they were different kinds of kids when they were growin' up. All's they wanted to do was eat and sleep here and move out as soon as possible. George and me tried everything to teach them how to love us, to teach them how important it was to be a family. They weren't interested," Liz said having more and more trouble getting the painful words out.

"Well, they're stupid," said Mark.

"Now, Mark-o, you know we don't like you to say that about anyone. It hurts me that they are the way they are and I'm glad you care so much about me you can see how much hurt they cause, but they're not stupid. They're just sad people who don't know how to love like you do," Liz said, trying to take the burden of failure away from her son and daughters. "Besides, maybe George and I had to learn our lessons with those three so we could become the perfect parents for you," she finished, emphasizing the word 'perfect' and smiling away her tears.

"Come here, big guy. That's enough sad talk on such a happy day. Come here and give Granny one last big kiss."

"Oh, brother!" Mark said as he kissed her. Liz could not help but wonder what the difference was. How could she have done such a poor job with her own children? What made them into selfish, uncaring people, uninterested in anything to do with family? Had she loved them enough?

****

I never thought the waiting would end. Just as I was beginning to think she'd never know I was here, she started to wake up. I sat by her side for five more days and nights before anything changed, then all at once I felt the familiar warmth creep back into her fingers and she squeezed my hand.

I gotta say the doctor, the one I thought was so casual about her condition, was right. She has been gettin' better since the last surgery. Her skin finished peeling and they say the yeast infection she had is gone. She's even been off the ventilator for short periods of time!

I knew she'd do it. I might have been having some doubts but in my heart I knew Liz wouldn't let something as ugly as cancer get her. I've begun to see that fighting spirit of hers, again. The nurse just told me they plan to get her up in a wheelchair this afternoon.

Welcome back, sweetie.

****

Chapter Three

It was Monday morning, Liz went about her kitchen duties while thinking of the wonderful Mother's Day she had. Mark's gift of roses, the breakfast in bed he and George had prepared and their leisurely day spent together. That Sunday together had been perfect. Even this quiet, routine morning was special. She loved getting up early and fixing a special breakfast for Mark. Putting the cereal on the burner to bubble softly, setting his place, watching the sun come in the windows as she went about her work brought a special joy to her heart.

"Morning, Granny," she heard Mark say as he entered her domain.

"Morning, Mark-o, sleep well?" She asked.

"Yup, how 'bout you?" he asked.

"Certainly did. I had a dream last night about a whole garden of yellow roses. I think your gift made me think of my father's garden and how beautiful it was. Thank-you again, sweetie pie."

"Granny, tell me about your father's garden. Will ya?"

She had to smile at Mark's sweet request.

"Let me get your breakfast on the table and I'd be happy to tell you," Liz said as she bustled around to serve her grandson his hot cereal.

As he started eating, she joined him at the table and began to tell of the glorious roses her father grew. She remembered what had seemed like a million different shades of yellow and gold growing in the small plot that was the family's backyard. Liz thought about her father's unceasing efforts to make their backyard a haven in the city.

"Mark, as long as I can remember, my father worked on that garden every minute he could. I can still picture him digging and pruning and dusting those flowers. He was as patient and loving towards them as he was towards our family.

We were so close. He taught me the importance of family and how each of us had the responsibility of caring for one another just like he cared for his roses and for us."

"That's how you learned to be such a good mother, right?" Mark said with a broad smile.

Liz knew he was exaggerating his sentiment a little, but she pretended not to notice. Instead she exaggerated right back and swooped down on Mark with a volley of kisses.

"That's right, my sweetie, that's right. Lucky for you that I'm the perfect mother!" She said between the smooches she planted all over his round little face.

"Oh, yuck, stooooop, okay, I get the point," Mark said as he started to laugh. "Too many kisses, that's one reason your not absolutely perfect," he said.

She could not resist tickling him just a little before sitting down and letting him finish his breakfast.

"I just want you to know how important family is, Mark. Do you know that when my father died, George almost demanded that my mother come to live with us. He said then and I know he still believes that family always sticks together."

"Was your mom all alone after your daddy died?" Mark asked with a somber tone in his voice.

"Yup, she was and my sister, Helen, couldn't see her way clear to take her in. George and I hadn't been married long, and mom was sick and I was expecting. My mother didn't have any money to help us take care of her. I never imagined George would want to take her in like that, but he did."

"What'd he say, Granny, I like to hear what he said."

"Well, let's see... I think his words were, 'Your mother doesn't have to live all by herself in that big house, I think she should move in with us.'"

"When'd he say it, Granny?" Mark asked.

"Right at the funeral, right in front of everybody and nobody asked him to. It was all on his own."

"Really?" asked Mark.

"Yup, really. And when I told him he didn't have to, he just looked at me and said, 'Yours, mine, who's ever. If family is in need, it's my way to do all I can. You should know that by now, honey.' he said. Well, Mark, if I didn't know it before then, I knew right at that moment that your George was about as perfect as any man can be." Liz finished with a little chuckle and Mark seemed to catch on.

"Well, I'm goin' be just like my George." Mark said as he got up from his chair and gave Liz a kiss, right on the mouth.

"I bet you will, Mark-o, I just bet you will." Liz said.

Liz had been looking forward to this Saturday night for weeks. It was weekend after Mother's Day, but she still felt like celebrating and a night at the VFW with George and their friends seemed like the perfect way to continue her happy mood.

This was her first chance to show off the beautiful sapphire ring she had received on Valentine's Day and she made a concerted effort, from the moment she entered the meeting hall, to make sure everyone saw it. She roamed from table to table exclaiming, "See what my two loves gave me!" as she quickly pushed her finger, with its decoration, so close to the viewers face it was almost up his or her nose.

After repeating the scenario more than a few times, she felt George's strong arm around her waist. He escorted her to a table and pulled out her chair. That' was when she felt the snap of an errant garter strap and saw her stocking begin to sag. Before she could rescue her dignity, she saw a fat, hairy hand reach for the broken strap at her feet.

"Frank Conner, don't you have anything better to do than grab at a married woman's clothes?" She said as she bent over her now partially dressed leg hoping to pull the prize from his hand. It was too late. Frank and his wife always sat at the Ostlund's table. They were good friends, but Frank was a tease and Liz knew he wouldn't be able to pass up the opportunity to give her a hard time.

In the best tradition of the VFW 'cootie club,' Frank yanked the strap from her tenuous grasp and stood, holding it high above his head and announcing to the entire universe, "Hey, I got Liz's garter strap." He then proudly pinned it to the red beret perched on his head.

"Better that then my bra strap," she shouted, hoping to drown the thunderous laughter his announcement had caused.

She looked around and saw that even George was laughing at the events and she was forced to admit, it was funny. Frank continued standing and laughing, his laughter dying only as he proposed a toast to her and her 'snapping girdle.'

The rest of the evening was more of a celebration. Liz drank her fill of martinis, visited with everyone she possibly could, and generally had a wonderful time. She loved every minute of it, even the garter strap incident, now that it was over.

Liz never went to bed without going down to Mark's basement bedroom to tuck him in. Even tonight, as late as it was and as tipsy as she felt navigating the basement steps, would be no different.

She leaned over his bed to kiss him quickly as he slept.

"Old lady," he surprised her by saying, "What'd'ya do, just get back from Mars?"

"Oh quit now and give your granny a kiss," she said, never flustered by his teasing words. She knew the "old lady," bit was his special way of telling her how much he loved her. She leaned closer to him to sneak one more kiss from his baby face.

He quickly laughed and hid his face beneath the pillow.

"You just watch, young man, someday I'll be gone and you'll be sorry you never kissed me more," she said as she tiptoed to the door.

She heard his voice say, "Never!" as she pulled his bedroom door closed. She was sure he could hear her laughing all the way up the stairs.

****

The day school recessed for the summer, the Ostlund's headed east for Cincinnati. It was a vacation Liz looked forward to all winter and she felt it began the minute they boarded the train in Billings.

George still worked part time as secretary for the railroad credit union. He had retired from his formal duties on the railroad after dedicating thirty years of his life to it. His pension and her work at the department store didn't bring in enough money to support themselves and Mark, so George kept working.

When he started this 'second career,' as he called it, Liz had worried that it was too much for her husband. He deserved a lazy and comfortable retirement. After seeing how much he looked forward to his afternoons with his cronies and this trip to the convention, she realized the job was good for George. <u>He never has been much for sitting around,</u> she thought as she listened to the clickety-clack of the railroad tracks as they sped towards their destination.

Liz took a sip from her glass of champagne and looked at George. He and Mark were poring over an issue of *National Geographic*. George had always had an avid interest in places, their history and the stories each place had to tell. He had tried to convey that interest to their own children, to no avail. Mark seemed to be the one who would carry George's passion on.

"When are we going to get there, Granny?" Mark said after about an hour.

"Got ants in your pants already, boy?" George laughed.

Then George held up his glass of champagne and encouraged Mark to lift his glass of grape juice, "To us, to our first big family adventure."

Liz joined them in the toast and felt the flush from the alcohol spread to the tips of her toes. She decided that the glow she felt was not just coming from the champagne. It was coming right from Mark and George. Their joy, their simple happiness enveloped her in a blanket of contentment.

****

The two and a half day trip seemed like a cozy dream. Liz felt suddenly jostled to alertness when the train pulled into the Cincinnati station and lurched to its stop.

"Now are we there, George? Huh, are we there now, Granny?" said Mark for the four thousandth time since they started the excursion.

"Yes, Mark, we're there." Liz said, "Now just wait a minute or two more, young man, before you go rushing out of here."

As she said it she stood and rushed for the door, saying, "bet I'll beat ya both."

She heard Mark say, "Hey, that's no fair," as she left the seats and headed for the train car door. <u>Freedom!</u> was all she thought as she jumped off the steps and onto the station platform.

She walked slowly through the crowds, breathing the different air of the Ohio valley. She hailed a taxi as soon as she reached the street side of the station and was inside it, her head poking through the window when she saw Mark and George traipsing out of the station weighted down with their load of suitcases.

"See Mark," she heard George say as they approached the cab, "She must think she's a queen or somethin', already and waiting." He smiled broadly at her as he plopped the luggage on the sidewalk.

"Your suitcases, m'lady."

"Yeah, Gramps, a queen," Mark echoed.

"Oh quit your complainin' and get in this cab," Liz laughed back at them. This queen wants to get a hot shower and get the vacation really started.

Mark's head whipped back and forth so fast during the ride to the hotel, Liz thought he'd end up with a headache. He's never seen such a big city, she thought as she tried to keep up with his questions.

"What's that building, Granny? How come there are so many cars? What's that policeman doin' in the middle of the street? Can I get somethin' to eat when we get to the hotel, huh, George, can I? I'm starvin'. How many taxis do they have in this place, huh, Granny? Does everybody in the city ride in a cab? Is that a river? Did ya ever see so many people in your life? Is Cincinnati bigger than any city?"

Liz eventually gave up trying to squeeze in the answers between his questions and Mark never seemed to notice. She thought she saw the cab driver shaking his head back and forth and she figured he was as overwhelmed with Mark's barrage as she was.

They arrived at their downtown hotel and disembarked. Mark stood on the sidewalk as George paid for the cab. His small head was tilted as far back as it could go without falling off.

"Wow, Granny! Wow, George! Look at this building. Have you ever seen such a huge building in your life? Do you think it reaches all the way to heaven? Are there clouds at the top of it? Do the angels look in the windows?"

"Listen, Mark-o, enough questions, let's go," said Liz as she grabbed a handful of Mark's sleeve to pull him along.

She sat and had a cigarette in the lobby as George checked them in. It was a beautiful, old hotel and she felt like a queen just sitting in the midst of such grandeur.

"All ready, sweetie," said George as he approached her, dangling the room key from his large fist.

"George, you didn't tell me how elegant this would be. It's a wonderful place," she said.

"Well, if you think this is nice, wait 'til you see the room," he answered.

They started towards the elevator as Liz said; "Now I hope you remembered I don't like heights. What floor are we on? You got us a room close to the ground, didn't you?"

As soon as she asked and they boarded the elevator, George said softly to the bellman, "Twelfth floor, please."

"Oh my god!" Liz managed to squeak as the elevator started and her stomach fell to her feet.

"You stupid shit!" she said, "Why in the sam-hill did you get us a room that damn high up? You know I'm terrified of heights!"

"Oh for christ's sake you're not goin' fall out of the room!" said George instantly.

She was instantly silenced and looked first at the bellman, who had a stupid grin on his face. He's certainly enjoying this! She thought.

She made a face at the man controlling the elevator and heard George and Mark burst into laughter. She joined them and thought the elevator was rocking, they were laughing so hard.

Mark joined in the ribbing by jabbing a skinny finger into Liz's side. "You're so funny, Sweetie," he said between guffaws.

"Oh yeah? How 'bout I just throw you and your grandfather off this elevator? Then we'll see if you like heights as much as I do."

The Ostlund's marched off the elevator at the twelfth floor with Mark still cackling.

The room was gorgeous; Liz had to admit George had made a good choice.

"Don't you dare open those shades," she shouted as the bellman deposited their luggage and went towards the windows. He turned right around and headed for the door. He did not look directly at Liz as he left, but she noticed his lips were pursed and his sides seemed to be shaking. She stood with her hands on her hips, daring him to let loose with another explosion of hilarity.

As soon as George closed the door behind him, they could all hear his mirthful roars.

"The room is very nice," Liz said, wanting to complement her husband but also hoping to let him know that he really pushed his luck by surprising with a bird's eye view.

"Now, Liz, no need to worry. I had them send up a few martinis. You have a couple, and then we'll open the drapes."

"You serve me then, old man and no more comments about my fear of heights!" She said, finally feeling as if she were back in control.

****

Their week in the exotic city of Cincinnati whizzed by. They tried a new restaurant with each meal and explored historical sites whenever George didn't have to be at a meeting.

It was an almost perfect week. The one exception being that King's Island Amusement Park was closed for annual refurbishing. Liz knew Mark had been looking forward to riding the famous roller coaster there. George had told him all about 'The Beast' and she came to suspect Mark had learned the explicit details of her one and only ride on the speeding monster. She heard George and Mark muttering behind her on one of their strolls through the city. She had been walking about ten steps in front of them. She heard George mimicking a high pitched screech when she turned to see him bending over to Mark, saying in mock hysteria,

"Oh, George, oh my God, oh, no! Get me out of here! No I can't do this! Oh, George, I'm gonna die. We're gonna die! Oh, get me outta here!"

As he finished his imitation of her he faked the act of throwing up and he and Mark broke into giggling fits.

"George Ostlund I am ashamed of you!" She said with enormous emphasis as she turned and began to walk briskly away from the two of them.

They scampered up behind her like naughty puppies.

"Aw, c'mon, Sweetie," the big one started. "Don't get mad, I was just telling how scared you were so that Mark would know that even someone as afraid as you were would live through 'The Beast.'" George said mischievously.

"Never mind, George Ostlund, if you want our grandson to laugh at his grandmother, well, than you just go on your own way and I'll go mine."

"Liz honey," George said as put his hands on her shoulders and turned her to face him. "I would never do anything to make Mark laugh at you."

Liz knew that statement was a close to a bald-faced lie as she had ever heard, but before she could let him know exactly what she thought of his nonsense, he leaned closer to her face and said,

"Besides honey, I didn't tell him the whole thing."

She knew what was coming and before he could say another word she sped off, "Don't you dare, George Ostlund!"

As she took her first steps from him, she heard him say,

"Honey, I never did tell him that you were so scared you wet your pants."

They were both laughing so hard she wouldn't have been surprised to turn and see them rolling on the city sidewalk.

She stopped and turned, realizing that it would do no good, at this point, to try to stop the two of them from enjoying her travails.

She looked at the two goofs they had become. She honestly did not know which of them was sillier, the old man or the child. She shrugged her shoulders and joined in their laughter.

****

After they boarded the train and settled in for the return trip, Mark sat next to Liz and said,

"Granny, this week is already over. When I'm in school it seems like the week lasts forever. What made this time, when I'm having fun, go by so fast? Why can't it be the other way around?"

Liz looked at him and said, "Get use to it, honey. Life will be like this forever and as you get older, each day will get faster and faster. That's why we try to teach you to enjoy each minute. The school minutes as much as the vacation minutes because when they're gone, they're gone and eventually they rush by just like the countryside we're rushing through right now. When you get to the last station in life, though, there's no return trip."

****

<u>Mark's in fourth grade this year,</u> Liz thought as she stood at the kitchen sink, drying the breakfast dishes. She wondered how long she'd be allowed to keep him. How long would it be before Albert and Nacole wanted him back?

<u>Oh, well, can't worry 'bout that 'til it happens.</u> She thought as George entered the kitchen for breakfast.

They both had to work today and Liz was planning to pick Mark up from school. She picked him up as often as she could. She wanted to spend as much time as possible with that little man who continuously stole her heart. Each day was a treasure, she knew and she cherished every one of them.

Tonight her sister, Helen, and Helen's husband, Ray, were coming for supper. Liz made sure the chicken was ready to pop into the oven upon her arrival from work. She had baked an apple pie early that morning and left it cooling on the counter. Helen and Ray were special visitors and she wanted everything perfect for their coming.

Liz had all she could do to keep Mark away from the pie when he came in from school.

"I'm gonna starve by the time they get here," he said plaintively.

"You'll live. Besides I've got a few cookies saved away that might help you get through 'til supper. That sound okay?" Liz asked.

"Great, cookies, point me to 'um," said Mark gleefully.

Liz loved to see his enthusiasm for food, her food. She felt a lot of pride in her ability to fill his tummy and see his smiles as he sampled her treats. <u>Must be a mothering thing, or somethin',</u> she thought as she served his cold milk and cookies, "with a kiss on top."

"Give me two, George," Ray said as they started their fourth hand of poker for the evening.

Mark sat quietly at the card table, his chair right next to George's. He always sat with them when they played cards. He seemed content to listen to the sounds of the game, the jokes that flew as the evening went on. He would often tell Liz that the best part about Helen and Ray coming over were the stories Ray and George told late in the evening. After a couple hours of poker and more than a couple of beers, the men would begin their reminiscence of depression era childhood, World War II adventures and life in general.

"Oh, geez-us!" George exclaimed as Ray snapped his full house down for all to see.

"How do you do it, you old dumb shit, you." George said, only probably half-kidding.

"Well, while you were busy talking about bein' such a war hero and all, I thought I'd just show you a thing or two!" Ray said with a broad grin.

Mark chimed in with, "Too bad shark, better luck next draw," as he poked his grandfather in the ribs.

"Yeah, you think that's funny, huh? Well, how funny do ya think it'd be if I paid him off in your next year's allowance?"

Liz watched as Mark's eyes got bigger than ever. He looked at George, who sat still and stone-faced, then he looked at Ray who did the same.

"Oh you two shits stop it right now. Don't worry, Mark, I'll protect you from those turkeys."

As she finished her defense, she pinched Mark's flushed cheeks.

"Awww, Mo...I'm mean Granny, quit it," he said.

He had slipped more and more frequently, calling her 'Mom,' instead of 'Granny' or 'Sweetie.' She knew it came from his heart and it endeared him to her more than ever. Liz also knew why he stopped mid-word and corrected himself. Mark had described a recent phone conversation with Lee Ann.

"She was really mad, Granny, when I called you, Mom, by accident," he said.

It took several long talks between the two of them before Mark felt better about things. Poor guy, some things must get mighty confusing for him, she thought.

She leaned over to him and gave him one of her famous sloppy kisses.

"Oh, yuck, what was that for, I wasn't doin' anything cute then," he said with pronounced disgust.

"You were just bein' you, Sweetie, just bein' you," she said as she realized once again how much she loved him.

****

It's Valentine's Day and I cannot wait to see her. I brought a huge bouquet of yellow roses, they're her favorites and I'm so anxious to see her smile when I bring them in to her.

It's kind of a bittersweet day, really. She's getting better, everyone agrees, but she's still hooked to that damn ventilator and I wish she were making better progress.

Seems like I always catch her at bath time. No matter what time I come the curtains are pulled and someone's washing her or doing some kind of treatment and I gotta wait more time till I can see her.

Today's no different. The curtains are pulled and something's going on behind them. Guess I'll wander out to the nurse's station and see what I can find out.

"Jerry, how are you? How's my granny today?"

"Hi, Mark. Did you see her yet?"

"Naw, they're in there doin' something. The curtains are pulled, as usual."

"Well, that's because Dr. Harvey's in there right now capping her trach."

I couldn't believe it! I actually jumped into the air and gave good ol' Jerry a high five. Capping her trach. That meant she was coming off the damn ventilator, at least for a while. It was a huge step towards getting her home, a huge step.

Finally, I'll get to hear her sweet voice again. The same tender voice that woke me each morning, that made each day the brightest. The voice I feared I'd never hear again. It might have been taken away from me for good.

I want to hear her giggle over some silly joke. I want to hear her boast of her prowess at the poker table and shout about some injustice she felt she needed to stand up for.

I know, now, I had taken that voice for granted, never appreciated all it meant.

I will never take one sound for granted again. I'll appreciate each moment, forever.

I've gotta let her know, somehow, how much she has meant to me. Gotta give her something, something special. I almost missed my chance. She almost left me without ever knowing how much I love her. The time's coming real soon. I've gotta find a way to tell her what she means to me.

"Jerry, can I get a phone hooked up in her room today?"

"Sure, I'll see to it. And, Mark, they're done in there. You can go in and see her now."

That walk, down the hall to her room, was a long one. She was sitting in the chair by her bed, waiting for me like a queen.

"Hi, love," I said as I bent down and put my arms around her. I could feel her tears on my cheeks and feel her frail body shake with silent sobs.

"It's okay, Sweetie, you're going to be okay," was all I could say.

Chapter Four

It was the day of their thirty-sixth wedding anniversary. April twenty-third, nineteen seventy. Who could have ever imagined she would be so lucky as to hold on to George for all these years. Liz silently counted her blessings as she cleaned up the breakfast dishes and anticipated the night's events.

It rained throughout the day, that soft, warm rain that only April can bring. Liz wasn't bothered by the rain; she knew the night and her celebration would be perfect no matter what the weather.

By evening, though, the rain had stopped and their dinner and dancing under the stars became a reality. Liz loved to dance and George made sure this anniversary was extra special. He booked a table at a restaurant with a twelve piece orchestra and a patio for dining and dancing. Liz told him he was wonderful for thinking of everything.

"I see that you even arranged for a full moon," she told him during their first dance of the evening.

"Oh, honey," Liz continued, "I can't wait 'til we celebrate our fiftieth anniversary. I don't ever want to lose you."

George pulled her closer and said, "I know we'll still be together then. I can't wait either, in a way. I just don't want the time to go by too quickly. I couldn't bear to be at the end of our time together."

Liz thought that was one of the sweetest things George had ever said to her. She was sure they'd be together for a long, long time. She said quickly, "Fiftieth or a hundred and fiftieth, you're not goin' to be able to get rid of me. I plan on bein' with you forever."

George, always the more practical, said simply, "You've got me as long as the Lord sees fit, that's for sure. God knows you and Mark need me and I plan to spend as much of forever taking care of you both."

Liz laid her head on her husband's shoulder. You're a good man, George Ostlund, and I'm a very lucky woman.

They danced until they could dance no more. The orchestra packed up as Liz made one last stop "to powder my nose." She knew the evening was still in its infancy. She and George rarely went home before breakfast on their nights out.

The next stop was the small bar where they spent many casual evenings. Pete was the owner and bartender, and he had told them, many times, that whenever they walked in he had a long night ahead of him.

It was a neighborhood bar, the kind that served family style dinners and catered to its long-standing patrons. Liz loved the familiarity of it. She always knew everyone in the place and spent time visiting with the locals and gossiping while drinking her martinis.

When she managed to quit talking to everyone else and join George at the table, she'd report the latest stories to him.

"Mrs. Johnson had her hysterectomy last week and her husband said he's sick and tired of waiting on her. Would you ever get tired of taking care of me if I were sick, George?" She asked.

"Honey, you know better than that. We've already been through a lot together. Albert's troubles, Lee Ann and Lisa's rebellion, I stuck with ya all the way then, didn't I?" George said as he smiled at her.

"Without a doubt, love, without a doubt. But ya know I've never been sick, really sick, ya know and I will be seventy before too long."

"Hush, now, woman, you're worryin' about nothin'," George answered as he took her hand.

"George, if I ever get really sick, and you get too tired of it and there's no hope, you know its okay to let me go. Honest." Liz said with all the seriousness she could muster after six hours of drinking.

"That's enough of that," George shot back sternly, "This isn't a night for discussin' that and you know I'll never let you go, no matter what! So, you better plan on workin' real hard to survive anything that comes along, you hear me. I don't ever want to be without you."

Liz felt a few tears run down her cheeks. She got up from the table and bent over to kiss her husband. She kissed him hard, on the mouth and said,

"I gotta go powder my nose."

****

"Granny," said Mark as he sat on her bed, watching her draw the last bit of red across her lips, "why do women do that? I mean what is lipstick s'posed to do anyway?"

Liz turned from the mirror and smiled at him, "Someday you'll know what it's for and nobody will have to tell you."

"Aw, Granny, that's not an answer."

"Well," she paused to think for a moment, "Lipstick is really for us, I mean women wear it for themselves. It makes us feel pretty and dressed up, kinda like when George shaves because he wants to look nice. And besides, if you kiss a guy when you have lipstick on, the mark stays with him awhile. It makes you harder to forget." She finishes with the mischievous grin he adored seeing on her face.

"Does it ever wear off?" Mark asked, wide-eyed and obviously intrigued.

"Nope," said Liz with a little laugh, "So if some guys foolin' around on his wife he better watch out for a gal with lipstick, he'd have a awful time explainin' it.

"Oh, Granny, now I know your just foolin' me."

She hugged Mark and patted his head with another laugh.

"I'm ready," she said, "Let's go, Mark-o."

They walked out of Liz's bedroom and got their coats on. Liz noticed George was already in the car, he honked the horn twice.

"Come on, love, sounds like the old man can't stand to wait for one of my biggest reddest kisses."

They were at the bowling alley in fifteen minutes.

Liz knew how much Mark enjoyed watching her bowl. He always chose to watch her team and often said, "Granny, you're a wild woman on the bowling alley!"

Maybe she was. She knew she had a habit of lofting the ball out on the lanes and if it missed the pocket, she would turn, stomp her foot and yell, "OHHHH Suuugar!"

She also, frequently wiggled and danced her way into position, before throwing. Sometimes she'd do a slow, seductive, hip-waving promenade towards her position. At other times she'd hop, or skip, or tango her way to her favorite spot. She always turned to look at the other team members just before her toss. She was only happy if she kept them in stitches with her antics.

This night was no different than the others. Liz was the queen of her team and she was well aware of the crown she held.

"Granny, too bad you lost tonight. You looked great out there," said Mark, on the drive home.

"Yeah, I heard you were up to your usual stuff," said George.

"Well, we lost fair and square, no doubt about it," said Liz, "No reason to feel bad, Mark. We all gave it our best and the other team did better."

"Yeah, but it's no fair! You bowled a two-eighty, almost a perfect game. That other team must'a been cheatin' or somethin'," Mark said.

"Now hold on young man," said Liz, hoping the disapproval in her voice came through loud and clear. "Part of playing any game or trying any sport is good sportsmanship. If you've done your best and got beat by a better team, there's no excuse for calling them cheaters. Mark-o, I've taught you better than this," Liz said softening her voice a little.

"You know we want you to grow up to be an honorable man, to understand the rules of life and one of the most important rules is to be a good sport. If you lose, you lose, no bellyachin' about it. You learn a lesson, decide how to do better next time and congratulate the winner. Got it," she ended emphatically.

"Yes, ma'am," Mark said quietly, then added, "I'm sure glad I have you and George to teach me. A kid doesn't get borned knowin' all this stuff ya know."

****

It was time for baseball, Liz looked forward to spring, but this year was special. Mark was in Little League and she loved every practice and every game. She and George spent several evenings a week and all day Saturday watching Mark play.

It was definitely a family affair.

She raced out of work, this Thursday afternoon, to catch the last hour of practice. There was a big game Saturday, against one of the team's bigger rivals, and Liz had no intention of missing a chance to see Mark get ready for the challenge.

"Come on, Mark-o, you can do it. Hit a big one for Granny!" She cried out enthusiastically upon her arrival at the field.   Mark was beginning his first time up at the plate. She had gotten there just in time.

She heard the crack of the bat as it made contact with the ball. It was up, over the head of the pitcher and past left field before she could take a breath.

Mark rounded the bases and came into home. She noticed a huge grin on his face as he slapped the hands of his teammates.

"I knew you could do it! Way to go, Mark-o!" She shouted.

She stood at her seat, clapping, and yelling for several moments. She heard others in the stand shouting with support, too.

"You did it, love, you gotta home run! Yeah, Mark!"

She was trying her best to out yell everyone, so that Mark would know how happy she was. As soon as he finished getting congratulations at the plate, he looked right at her and gave her his best grin. It was all the happiness she needed.

"What'd'ya think, Granny, can we beat those old Bobcats this weekend?" Asked Mark at supper that evening.

"I think, my love, you're a star and you can do anything you want to do. Did you tell George about your winning home run today?" Liz answered.

"Granny, it wasn't 'xactly the winning run," Mark said.

"It was too," Liz said indignantly, "your team won by only one run. I'm sure it was yours."

She heard George laugh.

"Well," George said between laughing and choking on his food, "He did tell me about it and I told him how very proud of him I am. I think, maybe, our private practice sessions are helping a little. What'd'ya think champ?"

"I'll say, Gramps, I did 'xactly what you told me to. I watched the ball and knew just where it was gonna hit the bat, then wammo! I did it."

"You're a real slugger, that's for sure," said Liz as she looked at both her 'men.' I'm so lucky, she thought.

They finished their dinner and George decided it would be a good idea if they practiced a little extra with the big game on Saturday. Liz watched them from the kitchen window, her George and her Mark, talking, throwing the ball and laughing together. She wondered why, for the hundredth time, Albert had never wanted to play catch with George, or join Little League, for that matter. She couldn't remember ever having so much fun with her own children as she had with Mark. I wonder

55

<u>where I went wrong with them,</u> she thought as she stayed glued to her spot in the window, trying never to miss even one second of the happiness that seemed to surround her grandson.

Saturday morning for the Ostlunds started at five-thirty. The big game was at eight and Liz wanted to make sure Mark's uniform was perfect, white as snow and pressed.

"I don't know any other boy who has to wear an ironed uniform," Mark pouted a little at his early morning breakfast.

"Mark-o, my love, I made sure I didn't make any creases in it, so no one will know I ironed it. I am just so proud of you; I wanted everyone to know how wonderful you are. When they see you running those bases in a uniform that gleams in the sunlight, they'll never forget you."

"Oh, Granny, I'll probably have it full of grass stains before the second inning."

"Still, sweetie, it'll shine right through the stains."

"Oh, Granny," Mark said again, but with a little smile. He got up from his chair at the table and came to her. He put his arms around her and hugged her long and hard. "You're the best Granny a boy ever had. Someday I'll be as good to you as you are to me. Someday I'm gonna give you somethin' that you'll never forget. I wanna give you somethin' for all you do for me."

Liz felt overcome with emotion.

"Watch out, boy, that lip of hers is goin' to town!" George said with a chuckle.

"Go on, the two of you. Get the stuff for the game. We got one to win against those old Bobcats," said Liz, ruffled by the attention they were giving her.

She got up from the table and headed to the bathroom to shed a few tears and then to 'fix her face' for the game. <u>I'm so lucky.</u> She thought as she blew her nose and wiped the tears away.

****

Mark poked his head over the car seat and asked, "How long 'til we get there?"

Liz had heard the same question at least ten times since they left the house, an hour ago.

"A while, Mark, now why don't you settle back and look at the scenery or somethin'. You know it takes a couple of hours to get to Great Falls. I told Helen and Ray to expect us around dinner time. I thought you were looking forward to our little trip? Try and enjoy the ride, will ya, for Gramps and Granny?" George said.

Liz knew her husband well enough to know he was probably running out of patience with their antsy, nine year old grandson and she knew Mark wasn't going to calm down for a minute. He was flying high since his team's win, last night, and he kept talking about the next game. <u>It'll be hard trying to contain him all week. Why do they have a seven day break right in the middle of Little League season?</u> She wondered.

"Look Mark, I'll teach ya how to make crackin' noises with your gum. That way next fall you can try and drive your teachers crazy. How's that sound?" Said Liz as she turned to face the back seat of the car and handed Mark a fresh piece of gum.

"Neat, Granny, what'd'ya do?" the suddenly intrigued boy asked.

"Well, it's like this, ya gotta chew real hard to make the gum soft first," said Liz as she looked at Mark. His little round cheeks were puffier than usual and his jaw was moving up and down so fast she thought he'd rupture something. The sight of him made her laugh loudly.

Liz laughed even louder when the gum flew out of Mark's mouth and landed in the front seat between her and George. "Oh, geez, Granny, you made me lose my concentration. Now I lost my gum!"

"Now, Mark,," she said, trying hard to compose herself. "That's not quite the way you do it, but it's an interesting trick."

With that, George started laughing, too. Then Mark started. The more Liz laughed, the more George laughed, and the harder Mark laughed. George was laughing so hard he stopped the car.

"Now, listen you two juveniles," he said between guffaws, "I would expect these kind of antics from Liz, but from you, Mark, I thought you were much more grown-up." With that statement, George started laughing again.

It took all of them several minutes before they could calm down and George could start the car again. Liz winked at Mark as George mumbled something about 'no fool like an old fool. She then resumed her gum-cracking training session with Mark.

Ray and Helen were waiting in the drive as they pulled up. Liz practically killed herself getting out of the car. She was in her sisters arms in a second.

"Oh, god, Helen, it seems like a year since I saw you!" She said.

"I know, honey, for me too," Helen answered. "Now where's that handsome grandson of yours, I need a big kiss!"

Liz turned to see Mark escaping from George's side of the car. He stood about twenty feet from Helen and gave her a timid wave.

"He's at that age, ya know, when they start not wanting to be kissed," Liz whispered to Helen.

"Nonsense," Helen said aloud, "I know he'll let his Aunt Helen plant a big one on one of those rosy cheeks."

She had Mark in her grasp before she finished her sentence. Liz noticed Mark grimacing as Helen did, indeed, 'plant a big one' on his cheek. <u>You can tell we're sisters. We both have to kiss and hug the little ones,</u> Liz thought.

Liz and Helen walked arm and arm into the house, talking as they walked.

"Do they ever stop, Gramps? Every time they're together all they do is talk," Mark said.

"I don't believe I've ever seen them quiet, how 'bout you Ray?" George retorted.

"Naw, never," he said with a loud laugh.

"That's enough, boys," Liz interrupted. "You boys just bring in the luggage and stop the philosophizing!"

Dinner that evening was a real treat. Liz loved being with her sister and it was nice to help someone prepare a meal instead of trying to cook everything by herself.

The women had steak and salad on the table by seven and the men had it polished off before seven-fifteen.

As Helen rose to start clearing the dishes, Mark said, "Oh boy now comes the fun part!"

"Mark knows what comes next. We're teachin'ya right boy, aren't we?" George said..

"I'll get the cards and the chips, Aunt Helen," Mark offered.

"You take the trash out first for your Aunt, then we'll start the game," said Liz.

"I bet my George and Granny are gonna beat the socks off ya," said Mark exuberantly.

"'Nuffa that," George grumbled slightly, "besides me and Ray thought we'd try and beat the girls, what'd'ya think Liz."

"You can try all ya want, old man, there's no way you're gonna beat us," Liz replied snappily.

The game was on and Liz was happy for the chance to show her husband just what she and Helen could do.

They were, of course, playing poker. Mark sat between the men and often rested his chin on the table. Liz looked over at him several times and winked. She did it whenever she was trying to bluff about her hand. She caught George watching her, several times, and her bluff seemed to pay off. She and Helen were sixty cents ahead after an hour.

As the evening wore on, Liz was drawn into conversation with Helen more and more. They reminisced about when they were little, about high school friends, and old beaus.

"Damn!" Said Liz, "How'd I let that get by me?"

"Granny, I think you were talking too much," said Mark.

"Hush, now, Mark-o, we weren't talking too much, I just missed an opportunity," Liz answered as she looked up from her cards into Mark's face. She saw him roll his eyes as if to say, "I'm sure, Granny."

Liz reminded him that if he wanted to watch he had to keep quiet. She hoped this would stem his insolence. No chance of that, though.

"Granny?" He asked, "Why do you and Aunt Helen always have to talk so much?"

"That's quite enough, Mark," Liz answered while trying hard to keep her mind on the game. <u>There's no way I'm lettin' those turkeys win.</u>

"He's right, ya know," George interjected, "Why, if you were playing in Vegas they woulda shot ya a half hour ago for talking so much."

"Oh, horse shit, you old thing," Liz answered. "Helen and I can talk all we want AND win the game."

<u>If he thinks he can bully me, well, he's got another thing comin' Liz</u> thought as she laid down a full house.

"Take that, buddy, and Hah!" Liz practically shouted.

Helen jumped up and gave her another big hug.

"You did it sister!" She said.

"We did it, us, women, HAH!" said Liz in gleeful triumph.

She smiled at George who could only sit and scratch his head. Ray looked as if he had been hit by a truck.

"Now, say it, go'on, tell me we can't talk and play cards at the same time," Liz added defiantly.

<u>Time went by much to fast,</u> considered Liz on the drive home, two days later. She and Helen had talked the entire time they were together, still Liz felt, they'd never be talked out. Even as she watched the scenery flash by, she was thinking of things she had forgotten to tell her sister.

Unpacking and catching up on the laundry kept Liz busy as soon as they got home. In fact the next few days were a whirl of activity for all of the Ostlunds. Liz was back to work, Mark had practice and the usual Saturday games and George was putting in a few extra hours at the credit union.

Only at Mark's practice or his games, did Liz feel as if she could relax. She hooted and hollered with the best of them as she watched her grandson become the star of the Billings Bulldogs.

At the end of July, Liz watched Mark's final game of the season. She briefly considered toning down her usual pacing, yelling, and cheering Mark on to victory, but only briefly. As soon as the little guy rounded home for his first run, she was up from her seat and shrieking, "Yeah Mark-o, that's the stuff! You got it! Hey, everybody, that's Mark Ostlund who just won the game for the Bulldogs! That's my grandson!"

She continued screaming through all nine innings and she felt it more than paid off. The Bulldogs won the championship and Mark-o scored the winning run.

The team and all the parents were treated to a victory dinner, that evening. Liz lost no time in telling each and every parent who her grandson was and how proud of him she was.

"Liz, sweetie," said George as he pulled her away from her tenth encounter with a parent, "Don't ya think ya oughta tone it down, just a bit. It was the whole team who won; we don't want Mark to get too big a head over this."

"Oh, hell, George," she replied quickly and with a smile, "I always congratulate the other kids, too, but George, blood is thicker than water and it was our grandson who made the win. I don't think I could ever be too proud of him."

George was silent. He smiled and kissed her gently on the cheek. She knew he agreed with her, probably even wished he could do what she was doing. I love you, George, she thought as she meandered towards another group of parents.

The morning after the big win, Liz got up extra early and started the waffles. She knew George had been preparing a surprise for Mark for weeks and today was the day he'd unveil his gift.

"Granny, George, Granny, come quick!" She heard her grandson's voice call.

George had been sitting at the table while she worked in the kitchen. He rose and followed her as they walked out into the living room.

"George, Granny, where'd this come from?" Mark asked as he stood in his summer pajamas facing the living room wall and the new oak trophy case.

Liz had to admit her husband had done a beautiful job of carving the case. He had ordered the glass panels specially made for the door and sides of it and it stood next to the television set, Mark's trophy gleaming inside.

"Where'd'ya think it came from, Mark-o," she said as she looked first at the small, surprised little boy then to her grinning husband.

"Gramps...I mean, George, you made this?" Mark asked.

"Sure did, made it just for you and for that trophy," George announced.

Mark walked over to the case and touched it gently, slowly running his hand over the wood.

"It's the most beautiful thing I ever saw." he exclaimed.

He stood for a few seconds then turned and took a flying leap into George's arms. Liz watched as Mark hugged George so tightly she thought she could see the veins stand out on his forehead.

George had leaned down to grab Mark as Mark ran towards him. Once the little guy was latched on, he lifted him off the ground and held him in his arms. Liz wondered if George was treasuring the moment as much as she was. She wondered if he was thinking how few of those delicious hugs ever came from their own son, Albert.

"I've got waffles," she said after the hug was over. "How 'bout a real celebration breakfast?"

****

That summer flew by for Liz. She treasured each moment she could spend with Mark. She loved watching him swim, seeing him help George cut the grass and work in the little wood shop in the cool basement. It was a treat to have him pitch an errant baseball into the barbecue grill or ride his bike, accidently, into her flower garden. She could never admonish him for those things; she felt she was lucky to have the chance to watch them happen.

It was August, time for the fair and all the noise and excitement the midway would bring. *He's ten this year, we've been bringing him here for four years, four summers and four winters. God, how the time has gone by. I suppose he won't be happy on the kiddie rides anymore,* she thought, god, *how I hate those big rides.*

Liz knew Mark had been looking forward, all summer, to the chance to ride the Octopus or the big roller coaster that rattled as much as a junk man's truck. She liked to wander slowly through the crowds, watching the people both on and off the rides. She never liked the rides.

"Come on, Granny, I wanna get going!" Mark shouted as he stood about ten feet in front of her, hands on hips.

Liz stood and looked at him, *Oh, go away,* she thought as terror grew in the pit of her stomach.

"I'll be there in a moment," she said, waving him on. Mark, however, was not to be ignored.

"Grannnnnny...," he whined, "You promised, besides you know George never will ride the rides and I can't go on alone and... well...you promised," he finished as he walked towards her and grabbed her arm.

"Okay, okay, I'm going. You don't have to pull me," she said.

"Better hurry, honey, or that boy's gonna have a nervous breakdown," said George with a chuckle. "You know I'd go, but the doctors tell me not to."

"Oh, bullshit, George," Liz retorted, "I think you made up that excuse just because you don't like rides either."

George smiled broadly at her. Liz made a face at him and followed Mark to her doom, the Octopus.

"See Granny, we're perfectly safe. They even give you straps to hold you down," Mark said as they sat and belted themselves into the awful little cars."

Liz couldn't answer him. The straps certainly didn't make her safe, nothing on a ride that whirled you around until you puked would ever make her feel safe.

It was starting, she could feel the rumble of the machinery beneath her feet. <u>Oh God, please don't let me die,</u> she thought.

The world whirled about her. She kept hearing some woman screaming. Every breath or so she'd try to remember to look at Mark, to make sure he was still beside her. At some point, she put one arm around his shoulder and squeezed him to her. She was terrified that he'd fly right out of the blasted thing. She heard the screaming, constant, now and shrill. Then she realized it was her own screams she was hearing. <u>I don't care if I wake the dead,</u> she thought quickly, <u>I'll scream all I want.</u>

Suddenly, the ride stopped. It was over, but it would take several minutes before the she could stand up. The midway was still circling around her at about one hundred miles an hour.

"See, Granny, wasn't that fun?" Mark asked as the ride attendant helped her to the ground.

Liz couldn't answer. She concentrated as hard as she could on getting away from the evil instrument of torture.

"Well, honey, did you enjoy it?" George asked.

"Oh, shut-up," was all Liz had to say.

"You're hair looks as if the birds used it as a nest," George continued. "C'mon, don't you think it was a little fun?"

"You just shut up or I'll...I'll...I'll shoot ya!" Liz was vehement and George seemed to back away. <u>Good, I hope he knows how mad I am!</u>

George took a step or so back, then walked towards Mark, bent towards the little guy's ear and whispered something. Liz watched almost daring them to say anything. They didn't. George simply took Mark's hand and started walking down the midway.

"We'll just walk on ahead. We don't want to upset you after such a horrible experience," George said with what seemed to be a somewhat mocking tone to his voice.

Liz felt her face get hot. "Oh you two, I suppose you can't wait to have a good laugh about this whole thing."

As she said that, she noticed the two of them with their hands over their mouths. Their attempts to hold in the guffaws failed and Liz knew she was lost. Her anger escaped her as soon as she watched Mark and George laughing so hard they looked like the apes at the zoo. They were laughing and pointing at her. Soon she was laughing too.

"Okay, what's so funny, you baboons?" She asked them.

"Nothing...honest... sweetie, not a thing," George stammered.

"Yeah, nothin'...Granny... I mean...'cept the time you rode the Octopus with George," Mark gasped between his hysterics.

"Oh, George, you didn't?" She said. "You did, you told him about me and you on the Octopus." Liz felt silliness overtake her. She and George had laughed about her first ride on the Octopus for years. "Oh, god, George, now what will my grandson think of me?" She asked as she let her own laughter flow.

"It's nothin' Granny, I used to pee my pants all the time, 'til I grew up some. Remember, you told me not to be embarrassed if it happened. Well, we don't care if you peed your pants on the Octopus. It was just an accident," Mark said loudly and firmly in the middle of a huge crowd.

Liz was momentarily dumbstruck. She looked at the crowd around her, maybe, they hadn't heard. As her eyes swept the people closest to her, she noticed they had their eyes on her skirt. They thought he was talking about her peeing her pants right now!

"Oh, god," Liz said quietly, "Kids sure do say some silly things." She grabbed Mark and George's arms and pulled them away.

"You two are too much for me!" She said as she dragged the two, still cackling, guys as far away from the spot as she could.

Chapter Five

Liz closed the front door after watching Mark walk to the end of the drive to meet his friends. I can't believe he's in seventh grade this year, the little poop! He doesn't want me drivin' him to school anymore, huh! Guess I can't really blame him. Guess maybe he is too old for that kinda stuff anymore.

He sure looks handsome, though, she thought after starting for the kitchen and the inevitable dishes awaiting her. She was proud of herself for letting him pick out his clothes and for not interfering with his choices. She was shocked that George hadn't said anything about a haircut. She liked Mark's dark brown hair the way it was, falling just to his shoulders. She thought it made his green-blue eyes sparkle even more. She knew George preferred the Marine standard haircut for boys. She was happy that he wasn't making a fuss.

Only trouble with him bein' so cute, is the girls that'll chase him, Liz considered as she started the morning dishes.

Liz left for work after doing the usual morning clean-up. She planned to take off early that day and prepare a special dinner as a "first day in junior high surprise."

Let's see, I'll make peach pie, "that'll be nine, ninety-eight, ma'am," Liz told a customer between thoughts of menu planning.

"Yes, I think we have it in blue," she said later to another customer looking for a new work shirt for her husband.

Liz found herself daydreaming about the different, little surprises she might make for Mark. She kept her daydreams to herself for the most part, until she started to ring up a customer who handed her a peach colored tee-shirt.

"That'll be five, ninety-five, for the peach pie," she said inadvertently. She felt her face get hot until the customer looked at her and started laughing.

"You tell me whenever there's any of your peach pie for sale here and I'll buy it in a minute!" Said the lady she was waiting on. It was one of the women she had competed against in the pie baking contest at the fair last summer.

Liz got out of work at one-thirty, just as she had planned. First stop was the grocery store and her favorite meat counter.

"This a special cut," asked Joe Markham, the butcher.

"Special as special can be. Mark's first day in junior high. Wanted to give him a treat tonight." Liz said proudly.

"Well, let me just see if I can find the roast that fits the occasion," the butcher answered back with a smile.

Liz beat Mark's arrival by a half hour, just enough time to get the meat in the oven and the table set.

"Hey, I'm home!" She heard him yell as the front door slammed. She had to force herself not to run to greet him. She wanted to respect Mark's recent yearnings 'to be more grown-up.'

"Hey, Granny, what's all this," he said as they met in the dining room.

"Hay's for horses, my precious, almost grown-up teenager; and, it's a surprise," Liz answered.

"What for?" he asked.

"For you. Thought you'd like to celebrate your first day as a real teen," she said.

She could see he was pleased. His eyes lit up his whole face.

<u>So different, you're so different than those other three. They would'a thought it was 'dumb.'</u>

"Granny, you're the best!" He said as he came over to her and gave her a hug.

Liz couldn't resist. She planted a big kiss right on his still-baby cheeks.

"Oh, Granny, you didn't have to go that far!" He said as he pulled away from her and wiped his face with the back of his hand.

Liz had to laugh at him. He was so adorable when he was frustrated with her.

As they sat at the dinner table, that evening, Mark told his story of the first day at the junior high school.

"Ya know, I was a little nervous at first. I walked in the door of that school and...and, well, I never saw such a big place with so many kids! It was different when we went during the summer to check it out, nobody was there. This morning there must'a been thousands of people," Mark said as he helped himself to more meat and potatoes.

Liz watched him through the entire meal. So different than Albert, or Lisa, or Lee Ann. They never told us anything.

"And, George, ya'know I got shop class this quarter. Will ya help me learn about some of your tools this weekend so I won't feel too dumb," said Mark.

Liz knew it would make George the happiest man on earth.

"Of course, I will Mark, but you've worked with me sometimes. I bet you know more than most kids," George said with a silly grin on his face.

"Ya really think so?" Mark asked between mouthfuls. "Ya know as scared as I was, I think I might just like this place after all."

****

This day was almost too perfect. Granny spent several hours off the respirator and spoke her first, raspy words in months. George looked as if he had seen a ghost when he walked in that afternoon. There sat the love of his life, the queen on her hospital chair throne, smiling joyfully at him.

"Oh, honey," he said quietly as he bent down to hug her just as I had done.

I can only hope that someday I find someone to love as much as George and

Granny love each other.

I was surprised at Granny's first conversation. "Give me ten bucks, tough guy," she said roughly.

"What'd'ya gonna do, old girl, run out on us and take a cab?" George asked jokingly.

"Just give it to me," she said adamantly.

He gave her a crisp ten dollar bill which she handed directly to me.

"Take this right now and go buy those nurses the biggest box of candy you can," Liz ordered with a smile.

That's Granny for you, the first words outta her mouth in months and she's takin' care of somebody else. I guess that's just one of the reasons I love her so much! I sure hope God's watchin' right now, hope he's writin' one more good deed done in Liz's book of Life.

Lisa and Lee Ann stopped today, too. They did a good job of trying to encourage Liz and even promised to help her get home as soon as possible. I could see how their caring and concern helped Liz realize she very well could go home someday soon. I'll keep reminding her of how much we need her there and give her more reasons to try hard to get well.

We got her back to bed in time for lunch and for the surprise I had been planning.

"What's that for?" She asked as a burly guy walked in and hooked up the phone at her bedside.

"Gotta surprise, Granny, hold on just a minute," I said as I dialed a number.

I handed her the phone as I said, "Here, talk to Helen. You two've got some catchin' up to do."

I saw the tears well up in her eyes as she said her first 'hello' in months.

As I left the room, in order to give her a few minutes of privacy, I heard her say, "Helen, I'm back and I'm rarin' to go!"

I knew, then, that she wasn't ready to give up, that she'd keep fighting 'til she was well.

It was the best Valentine's Day I had ever had.

****

"So Mark-o," Liz said after a backyard barbecue one summer evening, "What do you want for your birthday? I haven't gotten any of the usual clues and I gotta admit I'm at a loss."

She watched Mark's face and saw his eyes light up, was he happy she asked or being timid about saying what he really wanted?

"Well, um....let me see. I'd like a, um... a" Mark stuttered.

"A what," Liz almost hollered, pounding a fist on the table in the hopes of spooking it out of him.

"A guit, a...," he started, "A guitar," he said softly.

"A what? A guitar?" George chuckled.

Liz thought this might be coming. She knew Mark was constantly engrossed in the recent noise coming from a 'rock and roll' station on the radio. She had dreaded this moment.

"What'd'ya want with a guitar? What'd'ya gonna do with it?" She asked.

"Play it, maybe get a band together some day," he answered.

"I don't want some long-haired hippie grandson, that's for sure," Liz said. As soon as she said it, she knew she was wrong. She watched Mark's face fall.

"If the boy wants a guitar, we'll get him a guitar," George interjected. "He's gotta learn about life on his own, you can't control everything he does. We both know what a good boy he is and I know we can trust him to keep on being good."

Liz thought about it for a moment. George was usually as against the new 'rock and roll' uprising as much as she was. <u>If he's willing to let Mark have a guitar, he must have more faith in that boy than I do.</u> She felt a little ashamed of herself.

"Okay, Mark-o, I trust you and your Grandpa. I'm sorry if it sounded like I didn't have faith in you, in the values I know you've learned. I know in my heart you'll never turn into one of those 'flower-power' weirdoes'.

Mark jumped up from his chair and ran to her. His arms were around her neck in seconds.

"You'll never regret this, Granny, I promise," he said as he kissed her cheek. "I promise to write a song just for you, soon as I learn how," he said.

"Okay, okay," Liz said, "That's enough, you just remember where you came from Mr. Rock and Roll, that'll please me more than anything."

"I will, Granny. How could I ever forget all the things you and George have taught me?"

Mark rushed into the house explaining that he wanted to look at a catalogue and decide which guitar would be best. Liz and George stayed in the back yard watching the evening sky.

"Ya know, you can't smother him forever, sweetie," George said after Mark left. "Ya gotta let him decide things for himself more and more. Neither one of us will be around forever; we gotta make sure he's ready to make the right decisions for himself. We'll start out small, not the best guitar in the world, maybe this time. Who knows, honey, this may be just a passing phase and he won't even go on with it."

Liz looked at George and smiled. He was right, of course, but she saw today as the end of her special closeness with Mark, or the beginning of the end, anyway. He'd soon enough be out chasin' girls and playin' in a band. Would he desert her completely as Lee Ann, Lisa, and Albert had done? Only time would tell, she decided, only time will tell.

****

"Halloween already! Look Mark, check out the marquis at the VFW Hall, a Halloween costume party and dance. I wonder if I can get your Grandpa to take me." Liz asked Mark as they drove home from the music store one brisk October afternoon.

"Can you believe it's gonna be Halloween next week, Mark-o? I don't suppose you're goin' to a costume party this year; probably think you're too old for that kinda stuff, right?" Liz continued.

"Yeah, too old for dressin' up or not old enough, like you and George, right?" Mark said as he turned and smiled at her.

"You hush, now, young one," she quipped, "I suppose your right in a way, when you get to be my age you don't care too much what anybody says, you just wanna have as much fun as possible."

"Um..." Mark stuttered, "well, I wanna have fun, too, Granny," he said hesitantly.

"Wha'dya mean, Mark-o? What kinda fun are ya thinkin' of. I hope we've taught ya enough about the wrong kinda fun, drugs and such. You aren't gettin' any ideas about tryin' anything like that, are ya?"

"Naw, Granny, I know better than that! I haven't even seen anyone who's usin' drugs and I know, even if I did see it, I'd never wanna try it," Mark answered quickly.

"I still worry about the effect that rock and roll stuff is havin' on you. You've never seen anybody use anything like pot, or whatever else is popular now a'days?" Liz asked.

"Granny," Mark said, "You gotta trust me, I promised a long time ago that I wouldn't ever do anything to disappoint you or George. And, I know usin' drugs would probably hurt you guys as much as it would hurt me. I love you and I won't ever do anything that would hurt you, so pleeese, trust me, okay?"

"Gotcha, kiddo," Liz answered, "I won't worry anymore. You're a good boy, Mark-o, I love you too. Now that we have that all straightened out, what kinda fun are ya thinkin' of havin'?"

"Well..." Mark started again, "I...I asked a girl to the junior high Halloween dance. Wha'dya think of that?"

Liz was almost overcome with emotion. Today was another major milestone in Mark's life, and in hers. His first date and he told her about it first. She was happy for him and sad for herself at the same time. He was growing up so fast!

"Oh, Mark-o, you're... that's....Oh, I'm so happy for you." As she said it she bent over and gave him a huge kiss, ignoring the fact that she was driving down the highway at over sixty-five miles an hour.

"Hey, cut that out!" Mark said. "Watch out Granny, you and your kisses are gonna get us killed," he finished.

"I'll watch out where I'm goin' when I'm done kissin' my grandson," she said playfully.

"Okay, okay, enough is enough!" Mark said as Liz tried to plant one more kiss on his round cheek before he turned away."

"Okay, okay, mister, no need to honk!" she said as she straightened the car's direction to avoid hitting a car in the next lane. "Some people are so rude, they honk at the littlest things."

"You almost hit him, Granny. Better keep your eye on the road or I won't live 'til my first date." Mark said with a chuckle.

The rest of the ride home, Liz hammered Mark with questions. Who did he ask to the dance? What was she like? Did they have a lot in common? Did Liz know her? When had they met? And on and on and on....

Finally Mark said to her, "Granny, I'm not gonna marry her, I'm just goin' on a date."

Liz smiled at the thought of it and gave him a huge hug as they walked into the house together.

"My little Mark-o, all grown-up!" She said.

"Oh, geez!" was all he answered.

It was the night of the Halloween party at the VFW and the night of the junior high dance. Liz had spent the last week making herself a mouse costume. She made George a costume with hugely padded shoulders, tights, and a medieval looking tunic. She rented plasterer's stilts from the local hardware store and decided George would be a giant from a fairy tale. <u>Although at six feet three inches, he hardly needs the stilts,</u> she thought.

George complained bitterly about the tights.

"What are you trying to do to me, woman?" He said as he dressed that evening. "You'll look adorable! I always did like your legs," she kidded him. "It took me a week to find those in a big enough size, you better wear them."

Mark's date, Susan, lived down the street. She came over at seven and she and Mark were being picked up by one of the other parents. Liz watched as Susan and Mark tried hard to hold in their laughter when she and George made their entrance into the living room.

"You two just hush now or I'll never get this old man to go out in this get-up!" She said.

"I don't think you have to worry about making an impression, George, you're so big, no one can miss you," Mark said in an explosion of giggles.

"Just wait, son," George said, "someday you'll be married and have some woman dress you up in some god-awful costume and then I'll have the last laugh, just you wait and see."

Mark and Susan continued their good-natured ribbing until Liz checked her watch, "Oh, god, George it's nearly seven-thirty, we gotta go!"

"What time is your ride coming?" George asked.

"Not for another fifteen minutes. We wanted to be sure you kids got off okay before we went out," Mark said with obvious pleasure.

"Very funny, Mark-o," Liz said as she kissed her grandson and made sure her glued on mouse whiskers tickled him.

"Don't stay out too late and behave yourselves, now," Mark said as Liz and George went towards the front door.

Liz shouted, "Stodgy old stick in the muds, you young people just don't know how to have a good time!" as she scurried to the car.

"Oh, yes we do, we're going to have a riot watching you two trying to get into the car," Mark yelled back.

****

I had promised her, on Valentine's Day, I'd have her home for her birthday and I've been working so hard to see so that I can keep my promise to her.

She's fed up, literally fed up, with the damned pureed foods. Every meal is a struggle. She keeps telling me she wants a steak, a charcoal grilled, bloody on the inside, T-bone. I'd love to give it to her and god knows she needs the protein, but her stomach doesn't hold more than a teaspoon or two of the mush I've got to feed her, let alone a T-bone.

I really thought she was doing better. She's off the ventilator for almost two hours at a time. She's tired of the whole mess, though, I can see it in her eyes. They draw blood every two hours, she fights every mouthful of food, and refuses to let certain nurses touch her.

She's tired of being in prison, she said to me the other day. "It's just like a dungeon, no sunshine, no weather, no day or night, just a lot of people around torturing us inmates," she croaked at me.

I don't know if I could stand it. I don't know how she's put up with everything this long. I just know I want to get her home as soon as possible and I don't care how much food she throws at me, I'm going to make her eat and get stronger and come home.

It's the fifth of March. I've spent most of every day with Granny since she's been in the hospital. I keep thinking, each morning on my way in to see her that today will be the day she turns things around. Maybe today she'll be better.

I always make a stop in the waiting room; grab some coffee and the latest edition of the paper to take to her. I wonder why George and Helen are sitting there. The nurses must have chased them out of Liz's room while they practice more of their torture on her.

"Hi, what's up? How's Granny?" I asked.

George is looking at me kinda funny, like he doesn't know what to say.

"What's goin' on?" I asked, "Has something happened to Granny?" I really am not sure I want to know the answer.

"Mark," George says quietly as he puts his arm around my shoulders, "The doctors told us that Liz' last CT scan show the cancer has spread."

I want to scream. I want to die.

"What...How...When," I stutter.

George looks directly at me, then he bows his head and says, "They say she only has six months to live. They say we can take her home, still, if she gets a little stronger, but they say it's spread too much to do anything more."

What kind of world is this! Where is God, why would he let this happen to her, of all people? Doesn't he know she's suffered enough? Why her?

I gotta get out of here, gotta get some fresh air. All I can think of is her face and her trusting smile. I lied to her; I told her I'd get her home and keep her there forever. How can this happen?

    I turned from George and started running. I ran out of that awful place, away from the smell of disinfectant and the failed promises of cures. They couldn't cure her, they couldn't help her. They had lied, too. All the medicine in the world hadn't alleviated her suffering and now they were giving up. She would die and nothing I or the doctors did would stop that.

Chapter Six

<u>I'm sixty-seven this year,</u> Liz considered as she checked her rapidly graying hair in the mirror. <u>No wonder those jam sessions set my nerves on edge.</u>

She was trying to ignore the noise coming from the basement. It was, after all, better that Mark was at home with his friends. She could count on "the band" filling each afternoon with its hard, crashing rhythms. <u>At least I know where he is, I just wish they'd play a little more like Glenn Miller and little less like the rock and roll maniacs!</u>

George was sixty-one this year, Liz marveled at his youthful patience with Mark's new activity. He would always calm her down and convince her that they should enjoy Mark's joyful noise.

"I sure try," Liz said to George as she fixed their afternoon snack, "but, I do not understand his taste in music."

Their days had taken on a new routine. Liz always got home from work before Mark's bus dropped him at the corner. He almost always brought at least one friend home with him for some of her famous pie and a tall glass of milk. About four o'clock every afternoon, several more boys showed up and the music would begin.

Liz and George spent most of the time, from four until dinner, in the kitchen, as far away from the noise as possible. George would read the newspaper and Liz would start the preparations for dinner. She'd frequently drop whatever she had in her hands whenever a loud, amplified crash of cymbals or drum roll burst in on their privacy.

She'd laugh at herself for being so surprised at the strength of the sounds. Then, she'd pick up whatever she dropped and smile at George.

"If I didn't love him so much, George, I know I'd never be able to put up with it," she'd say.

On a Wednesday, about three-thirty, Liz stood at the kitchen sink peeling potatoes. She thought she heard the bus squeak to a stop. It was her signal to start for the front door to greet her grandson.

She opened the heavy, wooden door and rubbed the ice from the glass of the storm door. She spotted Mark right away. He was walking backwards towards the Ostlund driveway. It sounded as if he was yelling something. <u>Is that Mark yelling,</u> she wondered.

"Nigger!" she heard the word and couldn't believe it.

"Honky!" she heard another voice say.

"Nigger, nigger, nigger!" She heard Mark say again. She watched and was horrified to see Mark flip his middle finger up in a decided gesture of contempt.

"Mark Ostlund," she screamed as she opened the storm door, "Mark Ostlund you get in here this minute!" She could barely hold herself back, she wanted to run into the yard and grab him by the scruff of his fourteen year old neck and pull him into the house as fast and hard as she could.

Mark looked in her direction and must have realized who was yelling for him. She saw him put his head down immediately. He walked slowly towards the door.

She stood with the door open to the Montana winter. She looked across the street and saw another boy. He was black and small, maybe younger than Mark. How dare her grandson ever use that word for anyone?

Mark was three feet from the door when she began her tirade.

"How dare you! How dare you use that word?" She began.

"But, Granny..." he answered without raising his head.

"No buts, no nothin', young man! You march to your room and think about what you've done. I'm so angry with you I need time alone before I can calm down enough to be even civil!" She said as she pulled Mark's coat and hat off him.

"Ouch, you're pullin' my hair!" He cried as she grabbed his stocking cap.

"Don't you complain one bit! Don't you even think of complaining! Now, march, young man!"

She stood in the hall, shaking with her anger. She watched Mark shuffle to the basement door and start slowly down the steps to his room.

<u>I can't believe how mad I am! I hate being mad, but I will not tolerate that kind of talk from anyone, especially my grandson!</u>

Liz hung Mark's coat in the closet and closed the door to the basement. She went into the kitchen and heated the coffee. As she pulled a cup from the cupboard, she noticed her hands were still shaking. How would she teach him the gravity of his error? How could she show him how wrong he was? Where did he ever get the idea that using that word was ever okay?

She sat at the kitchen table and smoked several cigarettes before she felt calm enough to talk with him. She put the half-empty coffee cup in the sink and crushed out her third cigarette, then started for Mark's basement room.

His bedroom door was closed. Liz paused a moment, knocked and announced herself.

"Mark, I want to talk to you," she said.

There was no answer. Liz opened the door. Mark was sitting on his bed with his head down.

"Mark, Mark-o, where did you ever learn that word? What made you think it would ever be okay to say it?" She said. She had prepared a more careful, controlled speech before coming down to him, but those words flew out of her head the minute she entered the room. What she said was what most concerned her. She was confused. How could her Mark-o ever let that word come out of his mouth?

"Granny, the other kids always say that," he answered her.

"The other kids say it. If the other kids say you should jump in front of a car, would you say and do it too?" She asked.

"No, 'course not," he said, looking at her for the first time.

"What other kids say and do shouldn't matter. George and I have taught you right from wrong and what you said was wrong and you know it."

"I understand." Mark answered quietly.

"You do, huh? How could you think that just because other kids use foul language to hurt people that it was okay for you to do it? You were pretty convinced it was okay when you were yelling across the street. If you were that convinced a few minutes ago, how did I change your mind so fast?" She asked. She did not want him to simply comply with her request; she wanted him to see why what he did was so wrong.

"Uh, I dunno?" Mark said, obviously confused.

"Well, let me put it this way," Liz continued, "All the years George and I have taught you to try and never hurt another person. We've tried to teach you that skin color or religion doesn't have a thing to do with who a person is. We're all the same, all God's children. But, in two minutes you were willing to ignore all our years of teaching and do what other kids do, why? And, why do you say you understand, now. Seems like you kinda flip-flop real easy on your sense of right and wrong."

Mark sat looking at Liz for a moment or so. She could tell he was thinking about what she said, maybe trying to sort out the problem.

"Uh, Granny, I didn't think before I called him that name. But I sure thought about it when you stood at the door and yelled! You coulda melted the snow with your look, I thought there was fire comin' outa your eye you were so mad!"

Liz almost smiled at that answer. She held back, though, and put her hand on Mark's shoulder.

"That's okay that I let you know how angry I was. I had every right to be that mad, but I don't want you to only behave because I'm angry. I guess that's what I'm tryin' to get at. I want you to never use that name or any other foul, hurtful word because I want you to understand how it hurts people and how we can only stop some of the problems in the world when we stop hurtin' each other.

Does that make sense to you?"

"I think so, I mean; I never realized how much that might hurt someone. Where do words like that come from? How did we ever get started using them?"

Liz took a deep breath. He was starting to understand.

"I don't know how they got started, I only know that there are nasty words for just about every kind of person and they are all meant to hurt. Like I said, the only way to stop them from hurting is to stop using them," she said.

"Okay, Granny, I promise I'll never use that word or any other hurtful word, cross my heart," Mark said.

"That's a start, Mark-o. I'm gonna give you some time to think about it, too. You're grounded for a week. No band practice, no friends, no T.V., got it."

"Yes, Granny," he answered as he put his head down again.

"And," she added, "I want you to think of a way to apologize to that boy. You think about it and come up with something and there's no dinner till you do."

"Yes, Granny."

Liz hugged him, then, hoping he'd know that she still loved him with all her heart.

"We all have lessons to learn, Mark. I'd say this was a big one for you, but I know you can learn it well and learn how to treat everyone with the respect they deserve. Don't forget, love, we're all God's children."

She kissed the top of his head and left him to his thoughts. She was still shaking with fear as she warmed another cup of coffee and lit another cigarette. <u>I hope I did the right thing. I hope I made him see. I don't want him to turn out cruel or uncaring. I hope I taught him in time.</u>

Liz went back to her dinner preparations. Mark was on her mind the entire time. She was silently cheering him on, hoping he'd come up with an appropriate apology before dinner. She would hate having to sit through dinner without him. He's got to do it, then I'll know he's learned a lesson and I don't have to make him stay down there anymore.

George came home a few minutes before the roast was done. She met him at the door and told him what had happened. He told her he thought she did a perfect job in teaching Mark. He also put her mind at ease as he told her that every young boy does some things wrong. He said not to think that their teaching, over the years, had been in vain.

"Mark will do some things we don't agree with, but I know, once we help him see his error, he'll do his best to change," George said as he hugged his wife.

As Liz put the food on the table, she was afraid Mark wouldn't be up in time to share the meal. She had just turned to George to see if she should relax her discipline and let Mark eat, when she heard his footsteps on the basement stairs.

"Granny, Granny, I've got it, I did it," Mark said as he rushed into the dining room clutching a piece of paper.

"Slow down, son, let's see this," said George who was already seated.

George looked at the paper and then handed it to Liz.

"Here, Mother, see what you think of this."

Liz took the paper and sat at the table. She read it in a whisper.

"It's Time," she read and looked up at Mark.

"Can't we love one another?

Whose right is it to judge

The color, beliefs, or actions of others?

Whose right is it to judge?

God knows it's time to stop.

All of us must change.
For peace will only come to pass,
If we can feel another's pain.

A mother stands at her son's grave and asks,
Whose right was it to judge?
When will the killing stop and suffering end?
Whose right was it to judge?

God knows it's time to stop.
All of us must change.
For peace will only come to pass,
If we can feel another's pain.

The answer is quite simple, it must start with me.
I have no right to judge.
I will not repeat the past, the choice is mine, a new day dawns,
I have no right to judge.

God knows it's time to stop.
All of us must change.
For peace will only come to pass,
If we can feel another's pain.

"It's a song I wrote, Granny," said Mark after Liz read the last line.

"Mark, it's beautiful! How did you come up with such a beautiful thing and in so short a time?" Liz exclaimed.

"Easy, Granny, I just remembered all the things you said and tried to put everything into it. You really like it?"

"Like it? I love it!" said Liz, barely able to hold back her tears of joy. He did hear me, he did learn from us. Oh, thank-you God for helping him understand so well."

****

I was in the park for several hours, trying as hard as I could, to steel myself to face Granny and the future. Who would tell her that we had all failed to save her? How could we help her through this last, terrible time in her life? What could I ever say to her? I felt as if I had betrayed her, promised her things I could never accomplish. The questions and my guilt rolled around in my brain until I was dizzy. There seemed to be no answers.

It was late afternoon before I felt brave enough to walk back into that place, her torture chamber. The halls seemed to stretch endlessly. I had plenty of time to worry about how it would be to face her. George stood outside of her room. He nodded as I came by, put his hand on my shoulder and whispered, "She knows," as I entered her room.

She looked every bit the queen of her world. She sat regally, straight and strong, in the armchair beside her bed. I moved towards her and realized, for all my preparation, I was going to fall completely apart. I couldn't utter a word. All I could do was to lean over her and gather her small frame in my arms. I hugged her tightly and lifted her out of the chair. I sat, holding her like a child on my lap.

We sat together, her head on my shoulder, saying nothing, for a very long time.

****

It's almost here, the time's almost gone. Liz thought as she cleaned the house.

Albert and Nacole, Mark's parents, were back in the States. Albert had been reassigned to Fort Bragg in North Carolina and the whole family, including Mark's three sisters, were coming to Montana to pick up Mark.

It was the day she had dreaded for so long. She could not talk with George about her feelings, he had dreaded this day for as long as she had. They had always encouraged Mark to keep in touch with his family and to love them, even at a distance. Now, though, now she and George were expected to simply allow Albert and Nacole to waltz in after fourteen years and take their boy from them. Liz couldn't comprehend what that would be like.

Family, huh! Liz thought as she swept and dusted vehemently, I hoped they'd never try this. I'd hoped they'd never want to pull Mark away from all he's known. Now I can only hope they'll see how happy he is and leave him be.

Albert and Nacole were due to drive in at any time. Liz took a break from her anger and cleaning and sat on the couch, losing herself in memories of other family times, other confrontations.

It was Lisa's sixteenth birthday she remembered most vividly. Lisa and Lee Ann got into one of their frequent brawls and Lisa left, in the midst of the party with the words,

"I'll make you sorry you ever took Lee Ann's side in this. I hate you both and I'm never coming back!"

Liz had to shake her head to get rid of the memory of that day. What had the fight been about? Why did Lisa think she and George took Lee Ann's side? That's how those fights always happened, though, some small thing between the sisters and Lisa always feeling as if George and Liz had taken Lee Ann's side. That particular fight had been a bad one. It was the day Lisa left and never came back.

"Granny, Granny," Mark said with his hand on Liz's shoulder.

"Are you daydreaming, Granny? When are my mom and dad going to be here?"

"Any time, now, Mark-o, you gotta be a little patient. They've been driving for two days, so I don't know exactly when they'll be in. Kinda depends on the roads and such, you know what Montana is like to drive in during February. We'll just pray they're safe, not worry so much about their schedule, okay?"

"Okay, Granny, I was just wondering," Mark said as he sat down on the sofa next to Liz. "Are you nervous, Granny, I mean...? I am, kinda. I hope they like me."

"Oh, sweetie," Liz replied as she put her arm around him, "There's not anyone in this world who wouldn't like you, don't you know that."

Her tenderness seemed to calm him. She'd never admit to him that she was, indeed, nervous. She was scared to death that Albert and Nacole would like Mark so much they'd take him with them.

<u>Gotta face facts, ol'lady</u>, she thought, They<u> have every right to love him and want him home. I have no right to hope that they'll let me keep him, but....</u>

"Let's finish our cleaning, Mark-o, and they'll be here sooner than we think."

It was after two when Liz heard the honking of a car.

"They're here! They're here!" She yelled as she ran for the front door.

George and Mark followed more quietly, all three stood in the hall as Albert, Nacole, and the girls came through the door.

Liz noticed Albert's expression as he got the first glimpse of his son. She thought he looked as if he was going to have a stroke.

"Mark?" Albert said with a quiver in his voice, "Is this my son? My god, you're so grown up!"

"I'm fourteen, Dad," Mark answered.

"Well, Mom and Dad, looks like you've done a great job. You musta' fed him enough. Look at you, boy, you've grown into a man," Albert said, still obviously astonished.

"I'm your mother, Mark," Nacole said as she stood in the doorway, behind her husband.

Liz looked at Mark as Nacole spoke. He didn't smile or speak or grimace, there was absolutely no expression on his face to indicate how he was feeling.

Liz thought it was time to take the pressure off her grandson. She said, "Okay, okay, before we wear our Mark-o out with all the introductions let's get everyone in and comfy. Sound good?"

She was hoping to give him a little breathing space. She knew it was almost to much for one fourteen year old boy to bear, this quick introduction to parent's he had never known.

The adults gravitated to the dining room table. As they started to talk, they noticed that Mark and his sisters had taken places on the floor, by the table.

Liz watched the kids talking. Polly, the oldest, was eleven and taller than Mark. Cindy looked like Nacole and Pam, the youngest of the three looked just like Mark. Maybe he does belong with them, she thought, as she saw them sitting together, laughing and talking as if they had never been apart.

They stayed at the table and talked. Albert had lots of stories about life in Germany and Nacole piped in on occasion to give a woman's view of living on base in Europe.

"I know we've only talked with Mark on the phone before, but I feel I know him," Albert mentioned after glancing down at his son and daughters. "Mark, you told me, in your last letter, about that guitar of yours. I'm sure the girls would love to see it."

"Would ya," Mark asked his sisters who nodded their immediate approval. "Is it okay, Granny and George, if I take 'em down to my room and show 'em the guitar and everything?"

"Sure is, sweetie," Liz answered him.

The kids disappeared for an hour or so and the adults continued to catch up with each other's lives.

"Well, Nacole, how 'bout helping me with supper? I think we could all use a good meal," Liz said as she rose from her seat and started for the kitchen.

Mark told Liz and Nacole, after supper was done, that it was an "absolutely perfect dinner since two of the most special women in his life fixed it."

Liz had to smile at that comment. He had certainly learned to sweet-talk women, just like George.

The kids played cards all evening. The adults joined in for several hands and when nine o'clock rolled around everyone admitted it had been a long, wonderful day.

Liz helped Nacole get all the kids in bed. She noticed that Mark kissed his mother without even being asked. Liz was happy that he was affectionate; she just wished he wasn't so darned wonderful this one time.

All evening, Liz felt as if she were waiting for the other shoe to drop. Everyone had been as sweet and happy as if they were part of a television family. It had seemed almost too good and unnatural to Liz.

When the kids were tucked in, George fixed all the adults a cocktail. They stayed at the dining room table and as Liz took her first sip, she closed her eyes and made a wish. Please don't let them ask what I think they're going to ask.

As she swallowed, Albert spoke. "Dad, Mom, Nacole and I would like to take Mark with us to South Carolina and finish raising him. We have a lot of lost time to make up. We both feel we don't want to be separated from him any longer. What'dya think?"

Liz had dreaded this very moment for the past fourteen years. What do I think, what do you mean, what do I think? Can't you imagine what I think after caring for him all these years. You just waltz in here and want to take him away. Hmmf, what

<u>do I think?</u> Liz steamed silently as she stared at Albert.

George spoke first. "Kids, ya gotta give us a minute or two, I mean, we kind of expected that you were coming to ask us about taking him, but ya gotta understand, Mark is part of our family and has been for fifteen years. We can't decide anything in a short time."

George looked gray, tired, and sad, Liz thought. She couldn't imagine their life without Mark and she imagined George felt the same way. She felt like crying and she knew her lip must be quivering violently. How would she survive this?

"Mom, Mom, don't cry please," Nacole said as she left the room and came back with a box of tissues. "Here, take these."

Liz blew her nose and tried to collect her thoughts. She took a deep breath and said, "I know Mark loves your father and me. We have taken good care of him. We are a family. Can't you see that taking him from us, just as he's growing into manhood, might hurt more than it would help. I have been a mother to him and feel very much like his mother. Tearing him away from me, from us, would be just like tearing any child away from its parents. Can you see that?"

Neither Nacole or Albert spoke. They looked at George and Liz, then at each other.

"Dad, what do you think?" Albert asked George.

"I don't know, it's just too quick. I feel as if Mark is my son and having him go with you would be the same as him dying. I can't just be his parent one day and become a distant relative the next. Did you think either one of us could do that?"

"I want you both to know," said Nacole, "that Albert and I are more than happy at the fine job you've done in raising Mark. We just want to give him our love, too, on a full-time basis. We've been saving that love for lots of years and know now how stupid and young we were when we had him. We were too stupid to realize what we were giving up."

"I can understand," said Liz as she took Nacole's hand, "We understand, but we also want to do what is right for Mark."

"We do too, Mom," said Albert, "We do too!"

The air was still thick with unfinished thoughts. Liz felt as if she'd explode if she had to explain how she felt. <u>Can't they see? If they're so mature now and understand what being a parent is all about, can't they see how it would be if we lost him now?</u> She didn't have an answer for that question. She imagined George thinking the same things. Albert and Nacole spent their life making quick decisions they regretted later. Wasn't this one of those and if so, what would happen to Mark if they decided, after he came to live with them, that they had made another wrong decision. Maybe she could bring that up, if her temper cooled.

George stood up and grabbed a few of the empty glasses from the table. "Might as well clean up a bit. How 'bout we leave this lay til morning. Give your mother and me a chance to think; to consider what we think might be best for Mark. How does that sound?"

"I guess that would be okay," said Albert. "We did kinda just rush here and jump on you with the idea. We can wait a day or so, can't we, honey," he said putting his arm around Nacole.

Nacole only nodded, and then said, "I guess I'm really tired anyway. Might as well get some sleep. We'll all be clearer in the morning."

Liz felt a little relieved. She had one more night until the decision would be made, one more night for Mark-o to consider this his home. One more night she knew she would never sleep through.

Liz kissed Mark long and hard when she made her nightly visit to tuck him in. She made extra sure the blankets covered him, she smoothed his hair, kissed his small head, and touched his cheek before starting for the door. <u>This might be the last time I can ever tuck him in</u>, she thought as she turned and took a last look at her sleeping angel.

While the rest of the house slept, Liz held a private vigil. She listened to George's quiet snoring. <u>Poor guy, he's worn out with all of this.</u> He had listened to her cry from the moment they entered the bedroom. She cried while she brushed her teeth. She cried as hard as she tried to brush her hair that George took the brush from her. He began to brush it for her, in long soothing strokes, while listening to her weep.

He was sleeping and she was alone with her prayers. She had continued to cry and no longer tried to brush the tears from her cheeks. She cried freely and silently while she prayed.

<u>Lord</u>, she pleaded, <u>why are you doing this to me? Why did you give him to me just to let them take him away. God, he's the only thing I've done right in my life. I goofed up my own children's lives but I helped Mark, I've helped him to grow up good. He's my one success and its been so wonderful to love him and have him love me. Why, God? Why do you want to take him from me?</u>

Her prayers mingled with memories as the night wore on.

In the midst of remembering Mark's fifth birthday and his beautiful smile as he blew out the candles on his cake, Liz noticed the light in the room had changed. Morning was coming. Soon she would know whether Mark would still be hers.

Chapter Seven

She rested a while longer. She was not eager for this day to begin. She checked the bedside clock every few minutes. I'll get up at six, not a moment before. I wonder how long after that he'll still be here.

At six she rolled out of bed and dressed quietly in the dim midwinter light. She went directly to the kitchen. She wanted to keep busy, to try not to think about losing Mark today. She started a large pot of coffee and made a coffee cake. No reason we should go hungry. No reason for Mark to leave...The thought that she would soon be sending her beloved grandson away today crept into the corner of her mind. Mustn't think of that now, can't stand it. She went on with her preparations for breakfast.

"Mornin' Granny," she heard him say. She turned to face the kitchen doorway and saw him standing there. Oh, how will I ever live without him. What will I ever do.

She stood there, trying to memorize every wonderful inch of him.

"Well, do I get a kiss from my favorite Granny or not?" he said with a grin on his face.

"Oh, Mark-o, I love you so much," she said as she hugged him hard and kissed him over and over.

"Enough of that, Granny, enough kisses. I mean I love you and all but that's too much for any guy to stand."

"Oh, you," she said, to full of sorrow for many words.

"What's goin' on out here?" George's voice boomed as he came into the kitchen and put his arm around his wife.

"I let Granny kiss me once, and she went absolutely nuts," Mark said again, grinning while looking first at George, then at Liz.

"Enough of that, you're certainly not too big to be kissed!" Liz said with exaggerated indignation. "How dare you complain! I'm afraid you'll never be too big to be kissed, not in this house."

That thought stopped their playful exchange. They knew what today held for them.

"Now you go back to your room, young man, and get some sleep. It's only seven; I don't think you've ever been up this early on a Saturday. You'll be exhausted," Liz said to Mark knowing that as soon as Albert and Nacole got out of bed the discussion and arguing might start. She didn't want him to hear it.

"I gotta say this is a first, Granny, usually you're hollarin' at me to get up or else! How do I rate extra sleep today?" Mark questioned.

"I'm just worried about you gettin' enough sleep. Now you go on and don't give me a hard time when I'm bein' nice," Liz answered back with a forced smile. <u>The longer he sleeps, the longer I'll have him.</u>

George piped in, "If I were you I'd take advantage of this, Mark-o, it might be the last time you get such a chance.

He patted Mark on the shoulder and sat down at the kitchen table to read the paper.

Mark shrugged his shoulders and gave Liz a quick peck on the cheek. "Guess I'll take advantage of this craziness. Never liked gettin' up anyway."

He made his way to the basement door as Liz finished setting the dining room table for breakfast and set the coffee cake on the cupboard to cool.

"Hey, Mom, what'ya cookin'. Sure smells good," Albert said a few moments later as he entered the kitchen.

Liz sighed silently. <u>I'm glad I got Mark-o out of here, just in time, too.</u>

"Oh, Liz," Nacole came in behind Albert and said, "You didn't have to go to so much trouble. I'm afraid we've made a lot of work for you."

"Nonsense, I want to cook for my family. I love to do it. I only wish my family would come around more often, instead of when they just want something."

<u>There, I've said it. I don't care, it's how I feel and I'm tired of pussy-footin' around my feelings. Besides, they can't hurt me anymore than they have by wantin' to take Mark away.</u>

She noticed that Albert and Nacole were sitting at the table, staring at her.

"I don't care what you two think anymore, I gotta say what I gotta say," Liz started.

"You two waltz in here after years of infrequent phone calls and little support for that boy you want so much now. Where were you when he was sick with the flu or getting his first teeth or playing softball? You haven't mentioned why, all of a sudden, he's so precious to you. He wasn't precious enough for you to want him all these years, now you show up and say you can't live without him. Sorry if I'm not kinder, but I don't really understand."

"Well, Mom, it's like we said, we grew up and realized how much we missed with Mark, and how much we love him," Albert interjected.

"Bull-oney, pure one hundred percent nonsense," Liz continued.

You don't abandon a child for years, not caring one whit about how he's doin', if he has enough food or clothes, if he's growin' up the right way, then all of a sudden decide you love him so much. What's really goin' on?"

"Mom," Albert says quietly, "We were wrong, no doubt about it. You have done a beautiful job of raising Mark and we have done nothing. We were selfish and childish, but we did one thing right. We knew he'd be better off with you. You can't deny it, which was a good decision."

"Uh-hum," Liz mumbled.

"Why now, son," George asked, "Why do you want to disrupt his life so much at this point, besides hurtin' your mother after all she's done. Why would you do this?"

"We tried our best, George; to do what we thought was best for Mark. It was hard for us, too. We've missed him so much and we wanted to come to you to prove how much we've grown, how ready we are to care for him."

"Ya know," Nacole interrupted, "The most difficult thing a mother can do is admit she can't care for her own child. I did that and I did it after a lot of thinking and with years of questioning myself. Did I do right? Will my own son hate me for what I did? Did I give him to the right people? That's the only question that never bothered me much, I knew you'd be great parents for Mark. Now I want a chance to show him how much I've learned and how much I've always loved him."

Nacole's last statement touched Liz more than anything either of them had said before. She knew Albert and Nacole loved Mark and when her anger and fear cleared away a bit, she knew they had done more than call their son occasionally. They wrote, called fairly frequently and never forgot him on a birthday or holiday. She knew she had been unfair in some ways. She also knew Mark would be better off staying with her.

"What do you want us to say or do?" George asked while looking directly at Albert.

"Well, Dad," Albert said, "I'm glad we've all had a chance to air out the situation a little. Funny how we all beat the kids getting up this morning, although, I know I never slept last night and I imagine, Mom, you didn't either."

"No, I certainly didn't," Liz answered as she moved to the edge of her seat. <u>This is it; this is when they tell me they're taking Mark. This is the moment I've dreaded. Oh, God, I don't want to do this, help me live through this.</u>

"Well, it's like this," Albert continued, "We know how much Mark loves the both of you. We know how much you love him. Trouble is we love him just as much and hoped the day would come when we would be good enough parents to bring him home. It's taken longer than we wanted, but we want him to come home and we want your blessing."

That was all Liz could bear. She didn't know whether she'd faint or wet herself or just be violently ill right in front of everyone. She was going to lose him too. First, Albert turned from her, then the girls. Mark had been her redemption as a mother. He proved to her that she was a loving, caring person who could raise a child well. Now that the raising was finished, he'd leave her too.

"Mom, are you alright? Mom, mom," she heard Albert call. His voice brought her back from her thoughts and the overwhelming fear.

"Alright, how can I be alright?" she asked as she looked at her son. "You want to take away one of the only good things in my life. Do I have to get on my knees and beg you two? I will ya know, here let me show you how a mother can beg for her child!"

"Liz, honey, don't," George said as he put his arm around her shoulders.

"Don't tell me don't, George. I'm begging for my life. Albert, don't you see that Mark has been our life for as long as we've had him. He's proof that I can be a good mother, that I can love a child enough to show him how to love others. Why do you want to take that away from me? Have either of you considered what this will do to Mark? He's a teenager and being a teenager is tough. These are probably the roughest years of his life and you want to rip him away from everything and everyone he's ever known to satisfy your own needs. You are askin' for heartache. You'll take this good boy away and break his heart and expect him to be yours overnight. It doesn't happen that way. He'll only be confused and scared and angry and in the way of every teenager that ever lived. He'll deal with it by breaking rules, and laws, and your hearts. What will you do then, call us and say you've changed your minds. Ask us to take him back, broken and angry as he's bound to be."

"Mom, we have thought about it. We talked with a counselor at the high school near our home and he will see Mark on a regular basis to help him deal with these feelings. We don't want to hurt him any more than you do. We love him and have tried to make a home for him," Nacole said.

"Do you just plan to take him, will he have any say in this or are you planning to ask his opinion at all?" George asked.

"We're his parents," Albert said quickly, "We'd consider asking Mark how he feels about the move. I don't think we'd change our minds unless he was absolutely hysterical or horribly angry about the move. Let's face it, he's not gonna really be eager to come with us. You two have spoiled him like we'll never be able to. He's been an only child and he's had everything he could ever want. Coming with us may not be very appealing. He'll have his own room, of course, but he'll have to share our time and anything we can give him with his sisters. I don't think that would be any teenager's choice. I'd like to give him the chance to make the choice, but I know he'll choose to stay and I don't think that's best for him any longer."

"Not best for him, or for the two of you," Liz suggested with a deliberate tone of sarcasm. They feel guilty about letting Mark be here all these years and now they want to play real parents, huh! Not at the expense of my Mark-o, I'm afraid.

"Listen, Dad, Mom, we could fight this out in court, you might win, but I've consulted an attorney ..." Albert started, only to be quickly cut off by George.

"YOU HAVE WHAT?" George demanded.

"I con...consulted an...an attorney," Albert answered.

"Of all the low-down, stinkin' tricks! I can't believe it. You consulted an attorney. Well, that's just fine, boy. I'm glad you told me. Now we know what you're really all about."

"Now, Dad, don't jump to conclusions," Albert said.

"Don't you tell me what to do, not even for a minute. You listen to me. Your mother and I took Mark in to help you. We had no intention of spending our last year's raising more kids, especially when our own kids turned away from us. Do you know how hurt your mother has been all these years? You leave with little more than a thanks folks and I'll call ya sometime. Your sisters do the same. Do you have any idea of what that does to the mother of such children? Did we ever hesitate for one minute when you asked us to help, when you asked for money, when you asked me to raise your son? You didn't ask me to raise him 'til you were ready to be parents, you asked me to take care of him and to love him because you thought you'd never be capable of that kind of love. Do you remember that day, Albert? Don't seem like any lawyers were needed then. How dare you insult me and your mother in this way?"

"George, George, please, this hurts too much," Liz whispered to her husband. She raised the tone of her voice and looked at her son and daughter-in-law, "This is too hard. We're fightin' again and I just can't. I wanted Mark to know only love and that's what he's known 'til now. I don't want our lives to be destroyed by this. Albert and Nacole seem dead set on taking Mark. If I can't do anything about that then at least don't let him leave while we're all angry at each other. I don't want that to be his last memory of us."

Everyone at the table was quiet for a moment. George broke the silence.

"Okay, no more anger, but if you take the boy and don't even ask his opinion, Albert, I'll have nothin' to do with you from then on. Mark deserves to have some say, or at least think he has some say in where he lives. Will you please ask him and give him a day to think about it. If you must go against his wishes, he'll think you considered his opinion of some importance.

Albert and Nacole looked at each other, and then turned to George and Liz. They nodded. Albert said he'd ask Mark as soon as he got out of bed and that he'd tell him he had until the next day to make a decision.

Liz knew that what she'd always expected would come to pass. The only thing left for her to do was to protect Mark as much as possible, to make sure he started his new life without anger.

The first sleepy child roamed into the dining room soon after Albert and Nacole decided they'd ask Mark's opinion.

"Mornin' sleepy head," Liz said to her granddaughter, "How 'bout some of Grandma's special coffee cake and chocolate milk. That's the special when you come to Grandma's house, ya know, just for Grandma's special ones." She leaned over and pulled Cindy close to her. She needed that hug more than anything right now.

Mark slept through breakfast. When Liz got up from the table to start the dishes Albert announced he would go down to Mark's room, wake him, and "have a talk with him." Liz' heart fluttered but she said nothing. She continued clearing the table and started the dishes. <u>I won't think about it, I can't think about this. Oh, God help me.</u>

When dishes were finished. Liz helped Polly and Cindy with their snow suits and boots. The girls wanted to build snowmen and the day turned perfect for it. The sun was out, the sky bright blue, and the temperature in the twenties.

"It's a perfect day for snowmen ain't it Granny," Cindy asked as Liz struggled to get her boots on.

"My gosh girl, where did you get these big feet from," Liz asked as her face grew more and more purple while she tried to push the child's boot onto her foot."

"Daddy always says I look most like you, Granny," she said innocently.

Liz started laughing. She wore a size nine shoe, the biggest feet in the family. Cindy was right, her feet, at least, were just like Granny's.

The girls played outside until lunchtime. Albert and Nacole sat in the kitchen over long cups of coffee after Albert had his visit with Mark. Liz wished she had been a mouse in that room. She hoped her son had not tried to unfairly sway Mark-o, <u>I guess it's stupid to think he'd ever want to come to us permanently. These people are his folks, his parents. I'm really selfish to want to keep him away from them. I can't help it, if I'm selfish, God forgive me. I want him here.</u>

The day dragged on and on. Cindy and Polly fussed during the afternoon, "There's not enough to do here. Why aren't our favorite programs on? When can we leave?"

Liz found it hard to talk to either Albert or Nacole. She made lunch by herself, she wanted it that way. What could she say to these people, what could they possibly say to her? It was better if they were all quiet. Liz knew everyone must feel like a kettle about to boil over, <u>at least if we don't talk we won't be angry at each other. At least not yet.</u>

Liz knew that Mark stayed in his room since Albert talked with him. After she made lunch for everyone else, she prepared a tray for him and took it to the basement. She was curious as to how Mark was taking all of this and she couldn't bear the idea of him missing two meals in a row.

She knocked quietly at his bedroom door. "Mark, honey, Mark-o, I brought you some food. He didn't answer so she opened the door.

"Mark, Granny's here with some lunch for you." she said squinting in the darkness. The shades were down, the room light, off.

"How come you're sittin' in the dark, sweetie?" she asked.

"Granny...Granny..." he started. She heard him sniffling.

"You catchin' a cold, luv? Hope not, everyone in the house'll be sick."

"Naw, just a little sniffly," he answered.

She knew he'd never admit to crying. She'd never force him to.

"You okay, sweetie? I've been worryin' about all this decision makin' you gotta do. Kinda hard at your age, I imagine."

"Yeah, Granny, it's real hard. Can you help me, can you tell me what to do. I mean, I love you and George the most, but I love my parents too. Is that okay? I don't want to hurt you, but I don't want to hurt Albert and Nacole neither."

Liz' heart felt glad for his love and heavy for his need to choose. Life was never very fair.

"Listen, sweetie, George and I have done a real good job a'raisin' you. We know you'll do the best and right thing. Don't worry about hurtin' any of us. We all love you equal and we can be happy with any choice that is best for you, ya understand?"

"Are you sure, Granny? Will you love me no matter what?"

"Oh, my sweet Mark-o, I'd love ya no matter absolutely anything, ya got me. Don't you ever forget that as long as you live. Whatever your decision turns out to be, George and me, we'll be a part of your life forever. If you go to live with Albert and Nacole, we'll make sure you **come** visit all the time. You don't think we're gonna let you get away from us now do you?" She asked as her heart felt like it had split down the middle.

"Oh, Granny, thank-you, you're the best Granny in the whole wide world, ever."

"I love ya, Mark-o, that's all there is to it. If you truly love somebody, you always want them to be happy, no matter what."

They sat on Mark's bed, their arms around each other for a long time. Liz finally rose to leave. She placed her hand on her lips, kissed it and then placed it on Mark's forehead.

"Just remember we love you no matter what."

Liz could not believe she faced another night of torture. The only blessing this night held was that it had to be the last time she would lay awake through the long hours and wonder if Mark would continue to be hers. <u>Only tonight, then at least we'll know,</u> she thought at least a million times before six a.m. and rising to face a terrible future.

She made breakfast, again, and sipped coffee while smoking almost continuously. She had not even combed her hair or put on the always present red lipstick. She was too worn to put any pretense on how she was feeling.

"Sweetie, you look like hell," George said as he entered the kitchen a little before seven.

"That's the way I feel," she answered curtly. <u>No use in wastin' words. Don't want to think. Don't want to talk. Just want to get this day over with.</u>

She noticed George almost creeping out of the kitchen. He knew when to leave her alone and she was satisfied that she sent that message to him.

<u>How many more hours,</u> she thought as she mixed the batter for pancakes.

Albert and Nacole were up by seven thirty and Liz had to admit they looked as bad as she felt. <u>Do'em good to do some honest worryin'. Time they learned things don't always go the way you want the minute you want it.</u>

Albert spoke right away, "Listen, Ma, you know we gotta leave today. I gotta be back home by tomorrow and we gotta drive straight through to make it in time. We have to get Mark up and decidin' real soon.

"Are you still going to take him, no matter what his decision?" George asked.

"I think so," said Albert quietly.

"Don't understand all the pretending you aren't then. Don't you think that's kinda underhanded?" Liz added.

"We'll see, won't we?" Albert answered as he turned and walked away.

Nacole stayed in the kitchen, sipping coffee and not saying a word. Liz wondered what she might be thinking, what she thought of this family and of her husband. <u>Maybe she thinks just like he does, then we're in for it for sure.</u>

Liz went to the sink and started running water. She had to keep busy and washing dishes seemed like the perfect busywork.

The water ran, she squirted the soap in and watched the bubbles rise.

"Mornin' Granny," she heard Mark's sweet voice.

Here we go, she thought.

"Hi, sweetie," she said as she reached for him, for a hug, to feel him in her arms right that minute.

"Hi," he said as he kissed her quickly on the cheek.

"Where is everyone?" he asked.

"Oh, they're all around her someplace."

"I suppose they're all waitin' for me to make my decision, huh?"

"Well, Mark-o, I'd be lyin' if I said no, but, there's no reason we can't wait as long as you want us to. This is too important a decision. You take your time."

"Naw, Granny, enough waitin'. I made my decision and want to let everyone know what it is."

Liz planted a big kiss on Mark's cheek as the words left his mouth. "You're an angel, love," she said, "Now, go to it."

Mark left the kitchen and hollered for Albert and Nacole. Everyone gathered at the dining room table and as soon as they were seated, Mark said, "I know you've all been waitin' for me. Sorry it took so long, but I wanted to be sure to do the right thing."

Liz noticed Albert looking at Nacole. He took her hand and gave it a squeeze. *I just hope they love him as much as they say they will. I hope they love him as much as George and me.*

Mark continued. "I love you all equally, and no matter what I don't want you endin' up hatin' each other. Will you all promise me that won't happen? Huh, right now, promise me."

Liz heard George say it first, "I promise Mark, no problems. We will love you, Albert and Nacole no matter what." She followed his example, although she knew it would be much harder for her, "I promise, Mark." Liz heard Albert, and then Nacole repeat the promise.

Mark took a deep breath in and out before continuing. "I made a promise to God a long time ago. I can't tell you what it was, but I haven't done what I promised to do yet. Also, I know and love Granny and George. I know I'd get to love you and Nacole soon and I already do, some. But, I've lived my whole life here. I want to stay here in the winter for school and to spend time with Granny and George. I'd like to come visit Albert and Nacole in the summer, if that would be okay."

Liz couldn't contain herself. She jumped up from her seat, "Oh, geez, Mark-o," she said as she squeezed him tightly.

She felt happier than she had the day he was born. Happier than,...Liz suddenly remembered Albert's statement. He would take Mark no matter what his son's decision.

She looked at Albert. He was comforting Nacole who was crying. "Albert," Liz said, "Albert, what are you gonna do about this?"

"Give me a minute, Ma, would you!" He answered with an edge of anger in his voice.

Liz sat down quickly. <u>More waitin', I wonder what he's up to now.</u>

The dining room was absolutely quiet. Only George's resonant breathing could be heard. Liz felt the deep, regular; inspiration and expiration would quickly drive her crazy.

"Can't you stop that," she asked him in an angry whisper.

"Stop what?" he whispered back.

"That...that breathing!" She stammered. He simply rolled his eyes and continued to breathe.

Albert spoke, at last.

"I've been watchin' all of you, you three, I mean, over the last few days. I can that without a doubt you all love each other. You are a family.

I wanted that for us, too. I wanted my son back to be my son and to love me the way he loves you, Mom and George. Maybe he would in time; maybe he'd learn how much we really love him and how much we want to make up for all the years we've missed. But, maybe he'd just resent us, learn to hate us for abandoning him at first, then tearing him away from the folks who have been his parents all these years. I can't do that; I don't want that to happen."

"Albert, what are you saying, son," George asked quietly.

"Mark has shown me the true meaning of love. He is willing to give us the benefit of the doubt, to be part of our family for the summer. That's more than I had hoped for. I figured he'd come out fightin' mad this mornin' and demand to stay with you. Then I woulda been mad at everyone, mostly myself, and torn him outa here to prove I was the father. But he didn't do that and I respect him for it, respect what you did by teachin' him about love. He needs to be with his real family, you two. I hope he'll want to visit us, but I won't demand it."

Liz sat, her hand over her mouth, looking at her son. She was more proud of him today then she had ever been in her life. The years of worryin' were over. Mark was truly her own son and always would be. <u>Thank God, thank-you God, thank-you.</u>

Chapter Eight

"Come on, Granny, sweetie, come on drink one more swallow, then I won't bug you anymore, honest," I've been begging her for the last half hour to finish this liquid crap they say she has to drink. I can't stand the smell of it so I can't blame her for not wanting it, but she's going to blow away she's gettin' so skinny. I gotta get somethin' down her.

It's hard to believe she's still tryin' to get well. She is, even if she won't drink that awful smelly stuff. She exercises when they tell her too, even with tears pourin' down her face. She's always tryin' to cheer me up, always smilin' even when I know the pain is terrible. God, why do you let her go through this? She deserves to get well, she wants to get well but every time she's close you let some other problem get her.

She's back on the respirator again, at least most of the time. Her poor mouth and nose are so cracked and sore. At least they kept the trach in her throat so when she's unhooked and breathin' on her own she can eat and drink. I'm gonna bring her a big, thick milkshake tomorrow. I did it a week ago and she positively devoured it. Never told the doctors but it didn't seem to have any bad effect on her so I'm gonna start doin' it every day. Maybe that crap they give her is makin' her sick. It's certainly not helpin' things.

I also took it upon myself to get Lisa, Lee Ann and Albert up here. Yeah, they were all hearts and flowers with Granny's first operation, but they got tired of the constant visitin' and all and haven't sent a card or called in weeks. I let'em know just how their mother was doin' and that I thought they all should get their fannies in gear and come here and beg her forgiveness. Guess what?

They showed up. Oh, only for a day or so and not exactly begging forgiveness, but I think Granny is more at peace with the whole thing. I never will understand how those three came self-absorbed human beings came from such a dear, selfless lady.

"Come on, sweetie, I'll help you up in the chair. We've done this before and you need a little time off your back. Don't worry about the tube. I know how to move you. Won't it feel good to get up and move around a little? I'll comb your hair and give you your lipstick. You'll look great when George comes. Now you know I'm not kiddin', you look great to us any time we see ya sweetie. Don't you know that?"

It seems as if she gets less care now that they think she's not goin' to get well. I know they're busy here, but I wish they'd take a little more time with her, kinda get her fixed up. Oh, hell, they do all they can. I know that, I'm just gripin' to hear myself. I wonder if every family member of every patient does that. You just feel so out of control about everything. The only thing you can do is complain, put the blame on the doctors and nurses instead of the disease. No wonder people in health care burn out.

"There, Granny, you look beautiful and don't you dare roll your eyes at me."

"Hi,, George, how ya doin'?"

"Mornin' Mark-o, what time did you get here, it's is only eight a.m... You're gonna wear yourself out. How's my girl today? Give me a good kiss, will ya angel, I could use one this mornin'. I missed bein' beside you all night, ya know."

I noticed when George came she'd brighten up and she did. She does every time he's there; it's as if she saves all her energy so he won't know how sick she really is. I'm glad she does that, glad that she feels close enough to me to show her sickest, most cantankerous side to me, I'm honored by it.

"Hey, Granny, you loved that milkshake so much, I'm going to bring you another one, how 'bout that?" I asked her soon after George arrived. I figured they needed some time alone and she needed the calories.

"We gotta get some weight on you if you're goanna make it home for your birthday. We've only got a few more weeks."

She smiled and nodded at that. <u>Good, she's still tryin' to get home, that's the best thing I've heard in a long time.</u>

****

Liz got out of work early today. It was June and unusually hot, <u>can't wait to put my feet up and have a cold beer,</u> was her main thought during the drive home.

She jammed the transmission stick into park and whipped the car door open. <u>God would I love air-conditioning in this old beast,</u> she thought as she started for the front door and the cool interior of her home.

She stopped mid-step, "What in hell?" She spouted. The house should have been visibly rocking with the amount of noise coming from it. The deep BOOM, BOOM, BOOM seemed to rattle even the sidewalk.

She rushed to the door and as she opened it she realized, immediately what she was hearing. <u>Mark's band was practicing today, that's it. My, God, it's been over a year since they started, you'd think I'd get used to it.</u>

She tip-toed downstairs, hoping to listen without being noticed. After about three steps she realized the ridiculousness of trying to be quiet, <u>they wouldn't hear me if I drove a semi down here.</u>

They always set up the practice session in the large, unfinished part of the basement. She stood at the bottom of the stairs and behind the wall that divided that part of the basement from the finished section and Mark's bedroom. She heard her Mark-o singing. She knew his voice instantly. <u>He's good. He's really good,</u> she considered with pleasure.

The music ended and she heard Mark's voice shout, "That's it guys, for today. What'd 'a think, pretty good so far."

She heard another young male voice pipe up, "We need a little more work on that second section, but, yeah, I think we're doin' great."

She decided to let the boys know she was there. As she walked around the corner, Mark looked directly at her and blushed deeply.

"Hi, Granny,, what 'a doing' home so early?"

"Inventory was finished so I came home. You guys are really good, ya know. How'dya learn to play so well and Mark, how in the world did you learn how to sing like that?"

"Aw, Granny," Mark said as his blush rose again.

"Hey, thanks Grandma", one of the other boys blurted out.

She saw Mark glare at the boy, then say, "Hey, she's not your Grandma and don't you think you ought to ask her what she wants you to call her."

Liz smiled at her protective grandson, "Granny suits me best. You can all call me that if you want. I kind 'a like bein' everyone's Granny."

She wondered how Mark would accept that. He made her proud the minute he spoke.

"Thanks, Granny. Guess its okay, guys. I'll share her a little, but I can't say whether or not I'll share her famous apple pie."

"Nonsense, I made two last night Mark-o. There's plenty for all of you. Why don't you guys take a break and come have a piece."

"We're done for the day," Mark explained.

"Gosh, that's too bad, I know George would love to hear you and he'll be home soon. I don't care if you practice all night."

"Really," one of the boys said.

"Absolute truth,, cross my heart." Liz answered.

"You're right, Mark, she is great! I'm glad she's all of ours."

They polished off both apple pies and played hard until eight o'clock that evening. Liz surprised them with chili dogs, chips and lemonade about six and listened to the steady BOOM, BOOM, BOOM intently. She hid behind the basement wall several times to be able to hear the words and the melody. It was beautiful, they were beautiful. She cried silently and happily as she listened.

The song, I know Mark wrote it, it's as if he wrote it to someone he loved very deeply. I wonder who the lucky girl is. Oh, God, I hope he doesn't fall in love too early. Please let him have these years for fun and music and all before getting wrapped up in romance.

In bed that night, she asked George if they could talk a little before going to sleep.

"Of course, honey, what's on your mind?"

"Well, I listened a lot to Mark and his friends playing their songs. I think they're really good, do you? Or, am I just a grandmother who loves her boy so much I think everything he does is wonderful?"

"You are that kind of a grandmother, ya know," George answered, "but I gotta agree with you, they're pretty good. Where did Mark learn to sing like that? Nobody in your family is musical are they?"

"Nope,, nobody at all. And it's not like he's been in church choir or anything. Must be God-given talent, that's all there is to it."

"Must be," George added.

"Well, if we think they're good, don't you think other people would? I mean if Mark has a God-given talent, shouldn't we encourage him to use it?"

"Yeah, Sweetie, I think you're right, I mean, we might wanna find out if they're really good. I wonder if there's some way for other people, someone other than Granny and George, to decide if they really have talent."

"Wouldn't one way be to let them sing for an audience?" Liz questioned, "Couldn't we help them get a job singing somewhere, after more practice maybe and then see what the audience thinks?"

"Sounds pretty good, but I don't know if those kids are old enough to do all the things necessary to get a singing job and all that. Who could help them, d'ya think?" George said with a definite grin on his face.

"Me, of course," Liz proclaimed, "You knew all along what I was gettin' at, didn't you old man."

"Well, I kinda figured you'd be wantin' to do something to help that grandson of yours. Don't ask me how I knew, I just did."

"Oh, you," Liz said as she smiled at her husband and kissed him hard. "I love you George."

"I love you, too, Sweetie, now can I get some sleep?"

"You sure can," Liz said. She rolled over and knew she wouldn't sleep. She was going to be too busy figuring out how to make her Mark-o famous.

****

"Have a good day, my sweetie," she said to Mark as he left for school the next morning. She had plans for the day and for the first time, ever; she wanted him gone as soon as possible. She'd make her announcement at a special dinner. She could hardly wait.

Shopping came first. "I need the best roast beef you've got," she told the butcher at the market.

"Another celebration, Missus,," he asked with a wide smile.

"My boy's goin' into show business and I'm gonna help him get there. He's got talent, Joe, and I aim to see him be the star I know he was meant to be!"

"Well, we'll have to have the whole town celebrate if that happens, now, won't we," he suggested.

"Not if,, when!" She said very emphatically; <u>better to get these people</u>

thinking the right way from the start.

She made stops at the stationary store, "Give me the biggest banner you can make," she told the clerk at the counter, "I want it to say, 'Congratulations to Our Star' and be covered with stars and stuff, okay?"

"Fine with me," the dour-looking clerk mumbled.

"Oh, and can you have it done in forty-five minutes? I've got some errands to run and then I'll be back."

"Sure, lady," was all he said. His uninterested attitude didn't phase Liz one bit.

"And, by the way, someday you'll be able to say you met the one and only Mark Ostlund's grandmother. My boy's gonna be a star and you'll sure be sorry you didn't get his autograph or somethin' in a few years.

She left the store feeling like she had made it to heaven. I could always brag about him, but people just said I thought he was wonderful because he's my grandson. Soon, everyone will know how truly wonderful he is. Maybe by helping him reach the stars I can pay him back a little of what he's given to me.

She finished her other errands, got a new tablecloth, and picked up Mark's rhinestone studded jacket from the cleaners. She made it herself, in secret. Working after Mark was in bed in order to keep it a surprise. She had it professionally pressed and couldn't wait for Mark to see it. It had a big star made out of rhinestones on the back and little stars on each lapel. It was beautiful and she knew Mark would love it. He can wear it on stage, everyone who sings rock n'roll has somethin' like that.

She made one almost last stop at the Elks Club, the spot where she and George had spent so many fun evenings. Bill Bronson was sitting with his feet up on the desk of the office.

"Mornin' Bill," Liz said.

"Well, Lizzie dear, what brings you here at this time o'day, the bar's not even open yet," Bill said. He had teased her for years.

"Bill Bronson, you're lucky I don't haul off and smack you. Why in hell did I ever let you get away with callin' me 'Lizzie.'?"

"It's only 'cuz of our secret love affair, honey, you know that."

"And how's Alicia, Bill, still as busy as ever?"

"Oh, why'd you havta bring up marriage an all that," he said as he grinned. They had greeted each other the same way for the last ten years.

She started the conversation in earnest, then. She had set her mind to asking the Elks to have a dance for young people and for Mark's band to play. As the head Elk for this year, Bill could approve or disapprove her request. He never blinked an eye. Liz knew this would be Mark's first step towards stardom and she had helped him to it. She was thrilled and excitedly kissed Bill Bronson hard on his lips.

"Whooooa, now, Lizzie, ya know I only 'ben kiddin' all these years, don't you?" He said as he laughed.

"Gosh, Bill, I thought you only gave me the gig because of our love for each other." She laughed, too, batted her eyelashes with exaggeration and left with a decided and flirtatious sway to her walk.

The banner was finished on time. Her trip was a perfect success. She drove home, going eighty all the way and singing at the top of her voice. Someday, someone's gonna catch me, but not today, not today.

Liz baked and roasted, cleaned and cooked all afternoon. When

she was satisfied that everything was perfect, she stood quietly to survey her world.

Wrapped the jacket. Let's see, the cakes decorated and the table looks great. The new tablecloth sets it all off. He's gonna see the banner the moment he gets in. I can't wait.

George came home early, as Liz had planned. He surveyed her work and said, "You've done a great job, Liz. Is everything set?"

"Yep, can't wait to see his face." She answered.

Soon their waiting ended. "I heard it, the school bus, George, I just know it. Now come stand here under the banner and keep quiet. When he walks in don't say a word. Just wait and see what he says."

George smiled at her and walked to the dining room doorway where she had draped the banner. Mark would see it the moment he came in.

"Hey, I'm....." Mark said as he entered with his back to them and turned to see his grandparents standing in the hall.

"What's goin' on?" He asked. His eyes were wide with wonder and the smile on his face was quickly growing into a clown-size grin.

"You'll see as time goes on. This isn't the kind of surprise you get all at once, it comes little by little," Liz said with a giggle.

"Me,, a star?" Mark questioned as he read the banner.

"We know you will be, son, and we kinda wanted to help you on your way," George said.

"Now don't give too much away, George," Liz admonished. "I will let you in on the next part of the surprise, though, what's your favorite dinner?"

"Well," Mark thought for a moment, "You know, Granny, roast beef, whipped potatoes, and hot apple pie for desert. Is it, what we are have'n that for dinner?"

"The boy acts as if I never make it for him. Of course we are," Liz answered.

"You could make it a hundred times a month and I want it a hundred and one," Mark retorted.

"I thought so. Now, you go and do your homework and let me get that dinner on the table. The last and maybe the best part of the surprise come after your stomach's full."

"The best part of everything is being your son," Mark answered as he hugged both of them. "Someday I'll make you both proud of me, I'll give you something back for all the wonderful things you've done for me. I love you Granny and George."

He hugged them tighter for a moment. Liz felt her upper lip quivering and knew the tears were going to fall real soon.

"Go on now, get that homework done, sweetie. We'll call you. Dinner'll be a little early tonight, can't wait too long to see your face." She said as she patted his head and looked into his beautiful eyes. <u>Wish I could hold this moment still forever and ever.</u>

Dinner came early, as Liz promised. Mark commented on every dish.

"The potatoes are the best you've ever made, Granny. The roast is wonderful; I don't think I've ever tasted anything so good. Oh, Granny, this pie is delicious. Are these special apples or somethin'? How do you do it, you make everything so great!"

That was all he said, though. There was no real conversation. No description of his school day or talk of what the band was planning. He didn't have time. Liz had never seen him eat so heartily. The only thing he had to say in between mouthfuls was how good everything was.

When the last speck of potatoes, the last drip of gravy, and the last crumb of pie were carefully scraped from his plate, Mark sat back and let out a huge burp.

"Mark Ostlund, I've never heard such an awful thing," Liz said pretending to be offended.

"Aw, Granny, I was just let'n'ya know how good it was the way they do in some countries George heard about, right George?"

"That's right, um...I guess," George answered.

"I can imagine in any country, if any boy ever burped like that his mother would have something to say. Isn't that right George?"

"Um...yes, I guess that's right Sweetie," George said.

"Well, I guess it's time for the surprise," Liz announced as she glanced at

Mark. <u>He looks a little nervous, oh, goody, maybe he thinks he's really in trouble or somethin'. Bet he'd never guess what we're plannin'.</u>

Liz left the room to get her gift. George cleared a few of the dishes and sat down next to his grandson. Mark just sat and when Liz returned he still looked as if he didn't believe all this was happening or wasn't sure the surprise was a good thing.

Liz laid her carefully wrapped gift on the table.

"Is this for me," Mark asked.

"Sure is, you're the star of this family. We've always known it and you've certainly proved it lately," Liz answered.

"Yes, son," George continued, "We want you to know that we're here to support you in everything you do, but especially with your music. Ever since you wrote that song for us, we knew you had a calling, a special gift. We want you to practice as often as you can, here and, well, this is Liz's part..."

George was interrupted as Mark reached the inner wrappings of Liz' gift, "Oh, wow!" Was all he could say?

"Go ahead, put it on," Liz said as she directed him to stand and placed the jacket on his shoulders.

"You guys, how can I ever thank you. This will be great; I can't believe you did this all for me."

"Of course we did it for you, you're our boy and you know we love you more than anything," Liz said.

"I can never give enough back to you, not enough gifts or love or anything, nothing at all," Mark said as he stared at his reflection in the mirror over the dining room buffet.

"Don't need no giving back," Liz said firmly. "We love you and we want you to go as far as you can with your gift of music. George and I want to be your managers, help you get gigs, do all we can do to make you the star we know you'll be."

Mark sat silently at the table, jacket on, eyes shining. Liz continued, "You make words come out on paper better than anybody I've ever heard. You add those beautiful words to the sound of the music you write and it's always perfect. You'll go far and we want to help."

"Gosh, what can I say, except I love you both so much? "That's not quite all there is," Liz started.

"There's more?" Mark asked.

Liz knew by the look on his face and the way he squeaked out those words that he couldn't believe there could be any more to such a wonderful surprise. <u>Good, he's as flabbergasted as I wanted him to be.</u>

"Well, I talked with Mr. Bronson at the Elks Club."

"You talked with the manager of the Elks," Mark whispered.

"Sure did." Liz said, "And he can't wait to have your band play for a Halloween party the Elks are going to have for the kids whose parents are Elks. It's your first "gig!" I got that word right didn't I?"

"Oh, , Granny, Oh George!" was the only thing Mark said before the tears started rolling down his rounded cheeks. Liz had never seen him so overcome. He came quickly to her and buried his face in her shoulder. She heard him say, "I promise, Granny, I'll give you something so wonderful, some day, I'll make you so proud of me. I love you so much.

She knew she had done well, she was being the kind of mother she had always wanted to be. She was able to relax in her joy for the first time, ever. This moment was absolutely perfect.

June to October went by in a whirlwind of band practice and fun. Mark turned sixteen. Liz felt they had spent every possible moment during those months, together, the three of them. There were backyard suppers, weekend driving trips, and long lazy days of just being together. They had traveled to South Dakota, George's birthplace. She knew Mark learned a lot from hearing about George's early years and his life as a rancher's son. It was one of the best summers she could ever remember and it had definitely been too short.

****

Halloween and Mark's first professional appearance were tonight. <u>Another holiday, another milestone,</u> Liz considered. <u>his first professional appearance, life goes by so fast!</u>

The band had practiced every day since Mark's special dinner. All of the band members begged her to sit in on their sessions and offer comments. She did not tell them they were wonderful all the time, only occasionally. She was proud of herself for offering ideas and suggestions that really made a difference and helped them seem even more polished. She could hardly wait for this evening's performance.

"See ya at the Elks, Granny. Don't forget to get there at six thirty; I wanna run through the program one more time, with just you as the audience okay?" Mark said as he opened the front door to leave.

"Give me a kiss there Mark-o, one for good luck. I know you don't need it but I want one anyway and don't worry, I'm honored you want us to listen to your practice. We'll be there."

It went as well as she could have ever hoped for. The practice session was flawless. She promised to view the dance from the back of the room, since it was officially a teenage get-together. She stood at the back of the room trying to hold back the tears of joy, tears that would have embarrassed Mark. She felt so lucky to be able to be there, to watch from where no one could see her, to cry and laugh and enjoy the music and the lyrics that burned with Mark's love of life. <u>He is so special.</u>

This is such a wonderful night!

About halfway through the evening, Mark stopped the band and bent close to the main microphone. Liz wondered what he would say.

"Ladies and Gentlemen, I want to introduce my band to you and tell you a little about us and how we got started." He named each of the members and thanked them for their wonderful work, then he cleared his throat and said, "The band and I would like to thank the Elks lodge for giving us a chance. I, also, want to thank my parents, George and Liz Ostlund. Without their help and love I would have never become who I am. They taught me their strong values about earning your own way, about never giving up, and about how families have to love one another completely and support one another always. They are my heroes and I want to let the whole world know it."

Liz couldn't believe her ears. "Did you hear that George, he called us his parents?" She could feel the tears roll down her face. She didn't care. She loved him and tonight made all the years of work and worry worth it.

George stood next to her for most of the evening. He'd offer to get her something to drink, a chair, or to take her out for a breath of fresh air. She refused all of it and only wanted to watch this night, this one perfect night. She would watch so intensely that the images of it would never leave her heart. The night would be forever etched in her heart.

Chapter Nine

"Oh, Lizzie, honey, please don't cry, don't let them get to you that way," George said as he dabbed at her reddened eyes with his big cotton handkerchief and put his arm around her shoulder.

"You know I hate bein' called 'Lizzie,'" was all the response she could muster.

"Sorry, Sweetie, I know, it's just when you're so upset for so long...Well, no matter what I call you, you're really my pretty girl and I love ya. I hate seein' ya hurt so badly."

"Oh, honey, it seems like I've always been a problem for you, ever since you married me and decided to take all of us. We've been problems, problems, problems for you."

"Now, Lizzie," he said glaring at her, "and I don't care if you don't want to be called Lizzie, whenever you say somethin' like that you deserve it. We're in our sixties, for god's sake, don't you know by now that I love you and your problems?"

"Oh, George," she said as the tears started to flow again.

"Granny? George?" She heard Mark calling from the living room.

"You gotta go to him, George. Let me collect myself and I'll be right down to start dinner. Just give me a few moments, okay?"

"You sure you're alright, won't try and commit suicide or anything?" He asked with a wisp of a smile.

"Oh, you! Of course not, you silly old geezer. I'll get over it as soon as I can and get to what really matters, feeding my men their supper." She tried to smile at him through her sadness.

"See ya in a few, then, Sweetie." He said as he left and closed the bedroom door.

<u>Oh God, can you ever make this hurtin' stop? Will you please help my girls to</u>

know how much they hurt me and help them to stop?

Liz cried for a little while, washed her face, and then went towards the kitchen to start supper. She heard their voices and what she thought was the rattle of pots and pans as she reached the front hall.

"What in god's name is going on in here?" She asked as she entered her kingdom.

"Well, Granny," Mark started, "Me and George thought you needed a night off so we're cookin' and you're gonna be sittin'."

"What?" "I don't know how to sit! Are you men crazy?" She asked all in one breathe.

"No, Sweetie, we're not crazy, just worried about you and we know you need a night off. How 'bout if we all go to a show after dinner. It's dark and quiet, kinda, you know, romantic," George said as he winked at her.

"George Ostlund! We can't, the three of us go I mean, and be romantic. I couldn't anyway. Maybe the two of you," she said with a chuckle and a wicked grin directed right back at her lascivious husband.

"Hey, now, wait a minute. I have no intention of bein' romantic without you!" George bellowed.

"Granny, you know that," Mark said as he started laughing, "Listen if you two wanna be romantic I'd be the last one to get in your way. Besides, I might just have a date myself, how 'bout we double?"

"Oh, oh," was all the answer Liz could give. She felt better than she had in days. You two are so ridiculous and so funny. She thought, how can I stay in a sad mood with either one of you around?

"So be it," she said, "Let's double, you and your date keep an eye on us, we'll keep an eye on you. Sound fair?"

"Anything you say, Granny," Mark answered as he came close and gave her a hug. "You know we'd do anything at all to make you feel better, ya know."

"Oh, Mark-o, I know that, I really do. I guess I've been a real depressing person lately. I'm sorry. I don't want to take time away from us by feelin' sorry for myself. Do you forgive me?" Liz asked.

"Forgive you? There's nothing to forgive you for. It's those ungrateful daughters of yours!" Mark said loudly. "Why are they so mean to you Granny? Why do they keep callin' and makin' you cry like this? How could anyone do that to you?"

"They feel they're right in what they're doin' Mark. They've been told by the counselor they see that I was not a good parent to them. They say I drank too much and didn't really love them. Maybe I wasn't a good parent and now I gotta pay for it."

"Don't you ever say that?" Mark yelled. "You are the best Mother in the whole wide world. I can never repay you for all the love you've brought to me and I know you haven't changed that much from when Lisa and Lee Ann lived here. They're just crazy, that's all. They and their 'counselor,' none of 'em know what they're talkin' about."

"Now, Mark, you can't judge them. That's not our place. They got their own hurts and feelings' and such. We can't know how they decide what they do and I know 'em well enough to know they really believe what they're saying. I just gotta try and understand it."

"That's where I disagree," George piped in, "Liz, you can try to understand, but you can't take all the nonsense those girls dish out and think they're right. You forget, I was here for most of the time you raised 'em and I know what they're saying' is just plain lies. It's time I got on the phone when they call and tell them they should be apologizing to you and thanking you for all you did do, not blaming you for things you never did."

"You guys are so sweet and good to me," Liz said, throwing her arms around both of them. "You're all I need and it doesn't matter what the girls say, honest. I shouldn't'a let'em get to me like this when they get together and start their pity patter trip on me, it's hard not to feel like I was wrong and they're right."

"Granny, what got em started this time?" Mark asked.

"Oh, they heard about your band and that job I got you for Halloween. They said they tried to have a band and I stopped em and now I'm helpin' you. They say that proves what a drunken old fool I've become and they said someone oughta take you away from us, so you can have a proper upbringing."

"I never heard such a load of garbage," Mark said with a tone of anger to his voice that Liz had never heard before.

"You're right, Mark, its garbage. First off, the band they wanted to join was a band made up of kids that were known to use drugs. Your granny didn't want her girls involved in anything like that. Second, at the time, both Granny and I offered to help the girls start their own band, but they wanted everything at once, costumes and expensive equipment and they refused to play anywhere like the Elks, or church get-togethers. They've been angry ever since we told em we'd help em, but we could only do so much and we weren't let'n'em play any bars or lounges until they were twenty-one. As you can see, they never got over being' angry."

"Geez, Granny, I guess I kind of stirred things up when I decided to play in a band."

"Nonsense, Mark," Liz said emphatically, "your story is entirely different and you know it. You are a good boy who accepts what we can give and is thankful for it. You don't get involved in dangerous or illegal situations and you respect us and our values. It's entirely different."

"I'm sorry for them, Granny and George," Mark said, "They don't get to know you and love you like I do just because they're so blind to bein' good. They're blind to your goodness too. It's really too bad for them."

<u>Such deep thoughts for someone so young,</u> Liz considered.

"Thank-you, sweet,, sweet boy." She said to Mark. "I will always remember today and your thoughts. I love you so much."

"I love you too, Granny and you just wait, and when I get older I won't be callin' to holler at you or anything. I'm gonna do something so wonderful you'll get back all the love you ever gave to me, okay?"

"Oh, Mark-o," was all she said while she hugged him long and hard.

****

Liz sat in the living room. She had pulled her chair to the big bay window and opened the drapes. <u>The stars are especially beautiful tonight, I wonder if they are always so lovely on Christmas Eve.</u>

She guessed it must be approaching four in the morning. She had come out of the bedroom hours ago, wrapped in an old quilt, and wide awake. <u>I don't think not sleeping, is such a bad thing. I never felt so thoughtful, never really had the time to think in so much quiet. Maybe I should do this every once-in-a-while, just to put things back in perspective. I guess I can't be too sad that Lisa and Lee Ann aren't coming. Guess I can't expect them to get over themselves enough to visit for Christmas. I would a taken them in, though. It's not like Lisa said, "Mom, how can you say you want us when we've both told you how we feel about you?" I forgive them, even if they don't forgive me. I just still don't understand...maybe I never will.</u>

She sat, quietly praying and contemplating. She did not resolve anything, but by five-thirty she started feeling a little more peaceful. <u>Maybe I'm tired, maybe it's the Christmas spirit. I still have Mark. I know he loves me and I can't wait to see his eyes this morning when he opens up his present. He loves me and I adore him. I'm blessed with that. Some women don't have anyone to love them. I've got George,</u>

too. Why in hell am I sittin' here feelin' so sorry for myself!

She got up quickly, still wrapped in the quilt, and went back to her bed and George.

"Geez, woman, your feet are like blocks of ice! You been walkin' outside without your boots on?" He mumbled as she crawled in next to him.

"Nope, just sittin' and thinkin'. ...George?"

"What, Sweetie?"

"I love you. Merry Christmas," was all she said.

He turned and encircled her with his big arms. She was warm and safe and at least mostly happy.

"Grannnnnnny!" Mark screamed as he opened his gift that Christmas morning. "Granny ...George,, oh, gosh, Oh, Granny!" He kept repeating.

"I guess he likes it," George said as he smiled at Liz and took her hand.

"I kinda thought he would," Liz replied.

"Like it? Not just like it, LOVE it!" Mark said as he started to play the shiny, new guitar. "You guys are too good to me. This is the best guitar made anywhere. The amps are fantastic! It's everything I need to make the band perfect. You shouldn't'a spent so much money. Oh, Granny, oh George, I love it so much."

"Well, then we certainly shoulda spent that much, it's important for a star like you to have the best, right?" Liz said.

Mark carefully placed the guitar in its case and gave Liz and George a huge hug. Liz knew, by the light in his eyes and the way his voice squeaked when he tried to talk, how happy he was. This was really a Christmas to remember. She was so glad she had not allowed her grief over her daughters to overwhelm her. The quiet night of thinking and praying had helped. She knew she couldn't make her daughters love her or see that their version of the truth was wrong, but being with Mark and being able to enjoy him was the best Christmas present she had ever received.

She heard Mark playing his new guitar that evening. Liz sneaked downstairs to her favorite spot behind the wall and listened.

Mark sang, "Please know that this seed of love you've planted in me will never die"

She couldn't make out any more of the words, he was singing very softly, almost to himself. It sounded beautiful and she wondered if she'd ever hear the whole tune. She knew it would be one of the gifts this wonderful young man would give to the world. She couldn't imagine who he might be talking about as "planting" "the seed of love," but she was sure it would be wonderful.

****

Liz continued working at the department store through the winter even though George had been begging her to stop. He said that her age, the icy roads, and the speed at which she drove were a combination leading to disaster. He had been harassing, on this February morning, since they woke at six. After listening to the weather predictions for snow and sleet, he seemed more determined than ever and she had almost reached her boiling point.

"Lizzie, Sweetie, I know you're a good driver. I just know the roads are more treacherous than any driver can manage. I don't want you to die today or any day. Can't you understand that?"

"I know, I know," Liz answered impatiently; "I also know you think I drive like a maniac and that I'm getting too old to drive. Isn't that it more than the conditions of the road?"

"Wouldn't you want to be home with me a little more? Think of all the fun we could have," he said with a very wicked glint in his eye.

"Aw, c'mon, Sweetie, I don't want a battle today. I'm just worried about you and it's supposed to get icier by this afternoon. Can't I drive you into work?"

She looked at George and knew she'd have to give in. She was as worried about him as he was about her. <u>He's been having' those damn chest pains again and I've begged him about seein' the doctor. I just don't like him out in this cold weather. It seems to make'em start.</u>

She took a deep breath and looked at her husband again, "Tell you what. I'll allow you the privilege of driving me to work IF you let me warm up the car first and you cover your mouth with a scarf when we go out."

"Seems like a lot of nonsense to me," he said.

"I'm not kidding George, the last time you were out in this kind of cold you said it made your chest hurt. Oh, and one more thing..."

"For god's sake, Lizzie, I just wanna help you."

"I know, but I'm not lettin' you help me and have you gettin' a heart attack in the meantime."

"Okay, okay, what's your one more thing?"

"You got to see the doctor soon, within the next week and I'll even make the appointment for you."

"All this to make sure your safe! Oh, alright, I never do win an argument with you anyway, might as well not even try."

"That's right, Sweetie," she said brightly. <u>At least I won half way!</u> "That's what we got each other for, ya know, you keep me safe and I watch out after you.

She called the doctor's office for an appointment before she'd let George go out that morning. <u>We're not getting any younger and I don't want him to be the first to go. I know he'll do fine without me, but I'd never survive without seeing that big, old bear of a man lying beside me each night.</u>

****

I called Aunt Helen, George," I said as George came into the hospital waiting room that morning. "I just have a feeling Granny needs to see her sister and Helen was more than happy to come. I hope I did okay?" I asked.

It seemed as if I might have overstepped my bounds a little, but George looked worn out from all the caring for Liz. He knew how serious her condition was, even if the doctor softened his prognosis a bit when he talked with George. I had even called George's doctor and made him come and tell him how Liz was doing. Dr. Peterson had been more than a doctor, more like a friend to George and Liz for a lot of years. I wanted him to talk to George in plain English and leave at least a window of hope, something for George to believe in. He had to be the one to keep hope for Granny alive. I knew too much, and she was too sick to have any hope left.

George had been wonderful to Granny, every minute, and I know he still believes there's a chance for her to get well. He pushes her and himself because of that belief and that's exactly what she needs. But, he needs a break. I know if Helen is here for a while he'll be able to go home occasionally and rest more easily.

"Mark, that's a wonderful idea," he answered with a real smile, the first one I had seen on his face in many months.

"I know how much they love each other and if there's anything that will help Granny it's a visit from her sister. Remember when Helen and Ray would come for a visit and all'a you would play cards 'til dawn. You even let me stay up and watch."

"Do I remember? It seems like it just happened." George answered as he joined me on the waiting room sofa. "All's we could see was your eyes when you sat at the card table, but you had to sit in a big chair with 'no phone book, George!' We'd laugh and give you an old deck of cards to pretend play with but that only lasted a little while. You wanted to watch, 'the real game.' The first time we let you, you told everyone I had four queens. What a card player you were!"

"I think I still remember some of the really outrageous jokes Helen and Granny used to tell. Where'd they learn'em Grandpa? They were the kind of jokes a Marine might tell, but I don't think they were jokes most ladies would tell."

"Mark, that's an understatement if I ever heard one. I was a Marine and I never heard such stuff! That's your Granny, though, she's a fooler. Just when you think she's gotta be the most ladylike person you ever met, she tells a joke like that or flips her garter at ya. I think what she might be is a split personality," George said, laughing, "only she not only knows what her other self does, she eggs it on!"

I had to laugh, too. I pictured all the 'bad things' Granny was capable of and had to agree with George, there could be two parts to her personality. We loved both of them, though. We loved all of her.

****

Liz hung up the phone and turned towards the kitchen doorway to see Mark. <u>God, he's so grown up. Seventeen, soon, my little Mark-o will be seventeen soon.</u>

"Hi, Sweetie," she said just before she gave him a huge, sloppy kiss.

"Gosh, Granny," he said with a blush, "I love you and all that, can't we cut out a few of the kisses?"

"Nope, sorry, Mark-0, as long as you live here you is stuck with the kisses. Don't be glum, though, I'm sure I won't' be around that much longer.

"Don't even say that! You know I'm gonna live with you and George for a long time yet," he said suddenly putting his arms around her and squeezing, "I'll be glad to have kisses from my granny, too, honest. I was probably just tired and grumpy when I first came in, sorry, Sweetie."

"Mark-o, I was kidding and you have every right to say you don't want to be kissed by your grandmother any more. It happens to every mother and grandmother, the time comes when a girlfriend's kisses are the ones their sons and grandsons want, not theirs. I shouldn't have teased you. In all honesty, it would be too weird if you wanted sloppy kisses from me all your life."

"Granny, how do you always know what to say?" He said, looking obviously relieved.

"How was school today, love?" Liz asked, wanting to keep him talking, keep him with her a while longer. <u>I love this time of day so much! I don't know what I'll do when he's not coming home after school anymore.</u>

"It was okay, nothing spectacular. How was your day at work?"

Liz was in her glory. Mark used to go with her to the department store on some of her work days. He was about nine or ten the last time he "helped" Granny, but he always wanted to hear the gossip from the store.

"Well, I got a new young one startin' in the undies department. She's cute, Mark, maybe I should introduce you?"

"Never mind, Granny, I'll find my own girls if that's okay with you?"

"Sure, Sweetie never hurts to ask, though. Here see what you think of this." She said offering Mark a spoon with a bit of frosting on it. She was frosting a cake with a new frosting recipe.

"Ummm, what is it?"

"I call it "Chocolate Caramel Crème," do you like it, really?"

"I love it, you're one wonderful Granny, ya know. Tell me how work went. You started to tell me about the new girl, not that I care, but is she pretty?"

Liz laughed, "I thought you didn't want me to fix you up? Why would you care?"

"Never mind all that, just tell me is she pretty?"

"Yeah, she's pretty, but not too bright." Liz said to taunt him.

"Wha'dya mean, "not too bright?"

"Well, I was givin' her directions on unpacking the stock for her department ya know." Liz told Mark and looked at him as she finished the sentence. She wanted to draw this out, to make it one of her best stories.

"Yeah, you were telling her to unpack her stock, then what?"

"Well, she unpacked the girdles, slips, and panties, and arranged 'em real nice."

"Yuh, then what?" he asked with a little edge to his voice. <u>Good, I gottem really wondering,</u> Liz thought.

"Well, then I looked over everything and noticed something was missing. I asked her real plain like, 'honey, where's the flopper-stoppers?'"

"Oh, Granny, you didn't!" Mark groaned.

"I sure did, why shouldn't I? Ya gotta have flopper-stoppers, ya know, besides they're on sale!" Liz said and without lifting her head from her work. She couldn't help but smile to herself. Mark knew what flopper-stoppers were; it embarrassed him to no end to have her say that word.

"Anyway," Liz went on with mock indignity. "Anyways, as I was saying, I asked where the flopper-stoppers were and the poor girl stood with her mouth open. Can you imagine, alls I asked for was flopper-stoppers and she couldn't understand what I was sayin'."

"Granny, nobody except the people who know you know what flopper-stoppers are!" Mark said smiling.

<u>Good, he's startin' to see the humor in it!</u> Liz knew she was going to have him laughing soon.

"Anyways, she didn't know what I wanted. I had asked her kinda stern and boss-like so maybe that's why. I don't know for sure why, but she didn't even ask what I meant." Liz continued between peeks at Mark's ever-broadening smile and working on frosting her cake.

"What'd'ya do next to the poor girl?" Mark asked while obviously trying to hold back a giggle.

"Now I didn't do anything to her."

"Not yet, anyway," Mark said partially under his breath.

Liz looked at him quickly with a wicked grin, and then she went on with the story.

"Well, as I said, she just stood there. Then, she went over to the cupboards and displays and started opening doors and looking." Liz felt her lip quivering; she was going to explode in laughter just as she did in the store. "Well..." She went on trying to control herself," That poor girl pulled out every box, every girdle, every item from every cupboard in the whole department."

She noticed Mark was trying to hold his laughter in, he was unsuccessful, it burst out in a huge guffaw.

"What...what...happened next." He blurted out between chuckles.

"Well..." Liz started, also having a tough time controlling her laughter, "Well, that poor girl got all done looking and she stood in the middle of the department. She just stood there! Finally, I walked up to her. Her hair was kinda all over her head, she looked kinda flustered. I stood with my hands on my hips, trying to keep my boss face on and I said, 'Why, my dear, they were right here all the time.' I pointed to the huge box of brassieres sitting right in the middle of the floor. 'They're right here. Didn't you know what I meant, I mean everyone in the business knows bras are called flopper-stoppers, ya know, they stop the boobs from flip-floppin' all over."

By that time Liz was laughing loudly. Mark was bent over with laughter; neither of them could manage a word for minutes.

"Oh, Granny, you're cruel; I...mean...really," Mark stuttered.

"It was fun, really Mark, it was one of my best and I never even planned it!" Liz said while dabbing at the tears in her eyes.

"I still can't believe I carried it off, at one point Maggie from Linens came through and almost gave me away. I caught her and gave her a couple of winks while

Susy-Q was lookin' for flopper-stoppers..."

She started laughing again and Mark joined her. She knew it would take a while for either of them to recover. It was such a good story, she'd be sure to tell it whenever she had the chance. <u>Oh, god, I love to share a good story with my sweetie, oh, Mark, I love you so much.</u>

Chapter Ten

"I love our Friday nights at the movies, George," Liz said between mouthfuls of freshly made caramel corn. She always ushered autumn in with a batch. It was the first cold night in October. Mark was on his usual weekly date.

"I like them, too, Sweetie. Nothin' like sittin' and watchin' an old movie and eatin' caramel corn with you by my side. Nothin' better at all." George stated as he leaned over in his chair and gave Liz a kiss on the cheek. "Seems since that boy turned sixteen there's no keepin' Mark at home on Friday nights. Hasn't he dated every girl his age already? Who's he out with tonight?"

"Now, George, he just takes after me. You know I dated around a little in high school."

"A, …little?" George said, "a little…, why you were the subject of gossip from the time you were thirteen. A,… little? I've heard from most of your fellow classmates over the years and I can't imagine anyone nicknamed, "Lizzie the Lover," as having dated 'a little.'

"You big jerk, I never had that nickname and you know it!" Liz said playfully. "Okay, Buster, time for the secret weapon."

"No, Liz, not that, you know I can't stand it. I was only kidding, honest."

"Too,… late. You deserve a good tickle. You've been getting way too big for your britches and I'm gonna make you squirm.

With that, she attacked George with her fingers firmly planted under his arms.

"Oh...god....no.....Lizzie," he said between guffaws.

"No, not enough yet, tell me you made up that nickname. Come on, now, tell me or I'll keep it up forever."

"Please...stop," he said laughing and seemingly not ready to give in just yet.

"Ha-ha! Gotcha right where I want ya, big guy," she said still intent on his retraction.

"Okay...okay...you win." He said.

"Say it, say you made it up."

"I...made...it, Oh, god, Liz stop!" George said suddenly and very clearly.

She pulled her hands away quickly. George seemed to be getting blue. He was still breathing fast, in short gasps, even though she had stopped her assault.

"Liz, honey...I'm having so much pain...in...My...my chest."

"Oh, George, oh, I'm sorry! Oh, god, we gotta get you to the hospital!" She said as she watched her husband clutch at his chest. His face seemed to be getting bluer by the second.

Liz ran to get his coat and tried, unsuccessfully, to force his arms into the sleeves. She gave up and put the obstinate parka over his shoulders. She helped him off the couch and out to the car without stopping to grab a coat for herself. <u>No time to wait, gotta get him to the hospital. Don't wanna wait for some stupid ambulance either. I can get him there a helluva lot faster!</u>

George's head rested against the back of the seat, his eyes were closed. He looked as gray as the car upholstery. The only thing she could think of was to get him to the hospital as quickly as possible. The car was going eighty before she got on the expressway.

<u>God, it seems like this is taking hours. Oh, geez, George, please live, please be okay!</u>

She looked at him whenever she could. "George, George, answer me are you okay, honey, I know it hurts, just talk to me a little so I know your okay."

"I'm...okay," he answered weakly and added, "slow down a little Liz, I'm not gonna die today, honest.

"You bet you're not, big guy. I'm not gonna let you leave me and Mark, not yet. Besides, I'm the older one, I'm the one who's goin' first, remember."

George smiled a little at that statement. Liz realized she was sweating profusely, she felt as if she were having the biggest hot flash of all time. Just let me get him there. Please, let me get him there.

She soon saw the bright white cross on the top of the hospital. She could swear the beams of light from that cross were stretching out to draw her in. She was going to make it. George was gonna make it.

Ten minutes later she crashed into the cement post at the Emergency Room entrance. She threw the gear shift into park and without even turning the engine off, got out of the car, ran to George's side, and practically lifted him from his seat.

"Take it easy, girl, I'm still alive and there's no way you can carry me into the hospital," he said.

She knew her lip was quivering and that tears were imminent. "You let me worry about what I can do, okay."

He simply nodded and leaned against her. They made their way into the building. Liz began hollering for help the moment the doors opened, "Help, he's having a heart attack. Someone please help me!"

A man in white met them with a wheelchair and whisked George away with orders to Liz to "Stay in the waiting room until we call for you." She was too overcome with worry to protest.

She fell into the waiting room sofa and started to weep.

Please God, let him live, let him live. Don't take him away from me; I couldn't live alone without him. Please, please, please.

She kept her eyes glued to the hands of the clock. She was sure they never moved. She cried and paced and cried more. She felt as if she were having the heart attack, at the very least she knew her heart was breaking in half with the grief she felt.

"Excuse, me, please, excuse me," she spoke to a different man in white who entered the waiting room and was talking to another family.

"Can't you see I'm speaking with these people," he answered curtly.

"I know, I don't mean to bother you, but do you know anything about George Ostlund..."

He cut her off mid-sentence, "Listen, lady, I'm a doctor and caring for Mr. Remsen. I have nothing to do with Mr. Ostlund and I don't know anything about his condition."

"I'm sorry, I don't mean to bother you but is there someone..." Liz continued in the most quiet and demure voice she could muster. Part of her wanted to punch the guy, but she was so worn out, besides, George was always quiet and polite when seeking help. He always said best way to catch a fly was with honey. Maybe his way would work. Maybe she wouldn't have to yell and scream for help this time.

He interrupted her again, his eyebrows crinkled together, his voice was loud, angry, "Listen, I told you who I am and I do not wish to speak with you again."

Liz had had it. She had tried George's way, it hadn't worked for her. <u>To hell with nice!</u>

"Listen yourself you high-falutin' pill pusher, I asked nicely and my husband is just as important as Mr. whats-his-name here. You could have directed me to someone else, or you could have even told me to get lost in a much nicer way, but I will not be treated as some kind of bug, shooed off because I inconvenience you."

She could see through her anger and noticed the doctor was a young one, <u>Good thing he'll learn his lesson about how to treat people early in his career. He woulda turned out to be one more pompous son-of-a-bitch who thinks he bestows the blessings of his presence on whoever he treats.</u>

"I'm sorry, Mrs. who did you say you were?" He asked, still using a nose-in-the-air kind of voice.

"I'm Mrs. Ostlund, my husband is George. Will you tell me who I can talk to about his condition?"

"When I am through talking with the Remsen family I will take you to someone who can help and then, madam, I will have you thrown out of this waiting room for your wild and uncontrollable behavior."

"The hell you will, Dr. pain-in-the-butt," she said with a mock haughtiness to her voice, "Our doctor is Dr. Peterson. Do you know him?" Liz countered.

"The Chief of Staff,' the young doctor said with a sudden catch in his voice.

"Yes, sir, and now I will find my own way out of the waiting room and to my husband's side. If he has suffered anything while I've been trying to get information or help I'll be sure to let Dr. Peterson know. By the way," she said as she started towards the waiting room door, "Are you a resident here or an intern?"

"What?" he asked as if unable to believe she could have guessed.

"You heard me, what year are you?"

"I'm a first year resident," he answered blushing.

"I see," was all she said.

She walked to doors plastered with signs forbidding "Non-personnel" to enter.

"To hell with that, I'm goin' to see George." She said as she pushed the door open.

The room behind those doors was bursting with people, noise, and, from what Liz could discern, massive confusion. She walked from cubicle to cubicle, pulling the curtain aside and peeking in.

"Sorry, wrong room," she said to a man in the second patient area that was having some kind of red tube being placed into his penis. A young nurse had penis in hand and a major blush on her face when Liz interrupted.

"Ma'aam, you cannot peer into a patient's room, please, wait outside and I will come to help you," the nurse said quickly.

"How do you expect me to knock," Liz answered as she closed the curtain and walked to the next.

She softly called his name, "George, George," before pulling another curtain back.

"Liz, Lizzie," she heard his voice, she knew immediately he was alive. She took in a huge breath in relief.

"Oh, George," she said as she threw aside the curtain that blocked her view of her beloved George. "Oh, George, you're alive!"

"Of course I'm alive, where in the hell did ya think I'd be?"

She didn't know whether to slap him for being smart or kiss every inch of him.

"How...how do you feel?" She asked almost afraid to ask.

"I'm fine sweetie," he said quickly, "Hey; you're a great ambulance driver. If my heart attack didn't kill me you woulda!"

"Oh, George, you did have a heart attack!"

"Naw, no way, I was just kidding!"

"George, have you seen the doctor yet? Has Doc Peterson been in?"

"Yes, dear, I have been well taken care of. In fact, Dr. Peterson was on his way to see you? How'd you get back here anyway?"

"Not important at all," Liz replied.

Liz kissed George long and hard. Warmth flowed from his lips to hers and shot instantly to her toes. Was it her love for him, relief that he was alive, or just the letting go of the horrible anxiety of seeing her love hurt so terribly. She wasn't sure and she didn't care.

"Geez," she said as she broke from her kiss, "Whatever happened sure didn't affect your kissin' power.

He smiled and she brushed a few gray hairs back from his forehead.

"Well, I can see you made it back here, Liz." Dr. Peterson said as he entered the room and offered his hand.

She had always liked him. He had always been so kind to her.

She took his hand and he said, "Looks like George is safe, my dear, so you just stop your worrying and let us find out what really happened."

"You mean he didn't have a heart attack?" She asked quietly, afraid to say the word and make it true.

"No, no heart damage at all," the doctor answered, "I think he may have a small stomach ulcer that's causing all his pain. We'll take care of that very easily, a few pills and a little rest. How does that sound?"

"Oh, Doctor, you're wonderful!" Was the only thing she could think to say?

"Now, we've got to have some more blood work done and one more EKG, just to be sure. After that, as long as nothing new shows up, George can go home to your good care, say tomorrow afternoon? Sound alright?"

"Terrific," she said. Liz was so happy that George was going to live, she completely forgot about the incident with the young doctor. She was shocked when Dr. Peterson brought it up.

"Oh, by the way," the doctor said as he was leaving, "I've already talked with that rather stupid young resident you had the misfortune to meet. He'll be disciplined and I assure you nothing like that will happen again in my hospital. You folks take care now."

"What happened, Lizzie?" George asked.

"Oh, it was nothing too much. I'll tell you about it later. I just can't figure out how Dr. Peterson found out about it. He wasn't there and I never told a soul, yet. I had planned to though. God, George, he's a great doctor and you're a wonderful man!" She said, instantly full of the joy of knowing George was really alright. "I love you," she said as she started kissing him again."

"Careful, girl, remember I only get to go home if I don't have any more problems. Don't get me too worked up or that EKG'll be wackier than hell!" George said as he pretended to fend her off.

She gave him her best and broadest smile and dove towards him for a long, hot kiss.

****

"Mark's graduation was somethin', wasn't it?" George asked.

"Sure was! He looked so handsome in is cap and gown. I'm glad he got to play for the prom."

"That was your doin' Liz, he couldn't done it without you pushing' for him with the school board. You've been a great manager, Sweetie. I guess we could call you a pro. Think of it, you're a agent for a risin' star."

Liz felt a warm glow inside, spreading through her like the last rays of the sun that stretched over the evening landscape.

<u>I feel like a pro, but not so much a pro-agent, more a pro-mom. He's grown up. He's a wonderful man and I know I had a part in it. I helped him. I feel like I learned so much, did so much better than with my own kids."</u>

"He's a fine young man, Liz. We can sure be proud of him." George said.

"Did he tell ya he wants to "go on the road" by fall. What'd'ya think, George, is he too young?"

"Well, even if we think he is, we can't stop him at his age, shouldn't either ya know. We've done all we can for him and we've more than laid the groundwork for him to have a good life. We gotta trust him, I know we can."

"You're right, of course, old man. I think I'm facin' what they call "empty nest syndrome." I read about it in a magazine and it means that you feel bad about all the kids leaving' and the house bein' quiet and all."

"You didn't seem to have that feelin' when the girls left."

"Ya, I know, I didn't," Liz said as she pondered George's statement, "I didn't. There was so much heartache with those girls; it was almost a relief when they moved away. God forgive me for sayin' it., .almost a relief."

"Well, Sweetie, that's all over and the girls seem to be doin' fine, in their own way. I know you don't believe it, but you did a great job motherin' them two, they weren't the same kinda kids as Mark, that's all."

Liz smiled at her husband, not believing a word of what he said. "You're sweet, George, and I appreciate you saying that."

"But...," George said. Did he guess what she thinking?

"But, I still don't believe it; I don't feel I was a very good mother. I don't know if it was my age, or circumstances, or what. I wonder if I'll ever feel I've made up enough for my mistakes, but I appreciate you sayin' what you said."

George got up from his lounge chair, glanced up at the now starry sky and then bent over the seated Liz. He planted a kiss on her forehead. "You're a sweet lady and I'm an exceptionally lucky man, but you are way too hard on yourself. Mark didn't raise himself. He's all the proof of your mothering ability that you should need."

Liz looked up at George and felt more at peace than she had for a very long time. She could almost accept his statement, almost.

****

"I can't believe how much fun this is, isn't Granny? I never knew it would be this much fun." Mark hollered over the noise of the band music.

"Honey, you deserve this fun, it's what you've worked for and certainly what you earned. You guys sounded great. Now who is this playing? Have I ever heard of them before?" Liz asked.

"You probably haven't but everyone else from the Midwest to L.A. has, they're called "The Screaming Monkeys," Mark responded.

"I'll say," Liz said hardly able to hold in her laughter, "that's just what they sound like."

"Granny, we're the lead-in for "The Screaming Apes," can you believe it. I still can't believe you could do this, get us this gig!"

Liz could barely make out Mark's words. She was tired and ready for bed. She smiled at Mark and felt thrilled that this job had worked out for them, but she was feeling her age. "I think George and I will head back to the motel, honey. I'm glad you're happy, even though it's only one night. I was just sorry I couldn't get a longer spot for you."

"Granny the fact that you got us one night here, in Vegas, is terrific. No more bars and lounges for us. I just know it."

"Don't get too big for your britches, young man. There's no guarantee of success because of one night. Take your time, be happy for now.

"You're right, Granny. It's all because of you." Mark looked away from Liz for a moment. She could tell he was scanning the crowd, taking in the scene. They had finished their set just moments before and he was still flushed with the excitement of it. "Granny, is it okay if we stay for the main show and then get a cab to the motel, I promise we won't be too late. I just don't want to give this up yet. I wanna make the night last as long as possible."

"That's fine, Sweetie, not past one or two though, okay?"

"Gotcha, Granny. I'll see ya in the morning, then, okay?"

"Night, Sweetie, love ya." She said as she kissed him on the cheek.

Mark responded with kisses, first to her right cheek, then to her left. "Love ya lots, Granny."

Liz tapped on George's shoulder. He was standing next to her and Mark while watching the musicians now on stage. "Come on, big guy, I've had it for tonight. How 'bout you?"

"Yeah, I don't know how the kids do it, stay up this late and still have enough energy to dance around the way they do."

"George, honey, they're kids, that's how they do it."

George nodded his agreement and they started towards the door. <u>This has been great! Mark's band played beautifully. I think they're better than those Screaming whatsis anytime. Who could know that the owner of this place was an Elk. Thank god for Bill Bronson.</u>

"Well, Mark, turn and take your last look at Vegas," George suggested as they pulled out of town the next day.

"I know it's not my last look, I bet you anything I'll be back inside of a year to play more than one night."

"You're certainly full of yourself this morning, young man," Liz said. "Did you enjoy your night of stardom?"

"Are you kidding, Granny?'Enjoy' doesn't half cover it. It was wonderful and I loved every minute of it."

"Be sure and send Mr. Bronson a thank-you card, maybe have all the guys in the band sign it. By the way, we coulda driven another one or two of your band members home with us. Did they have other plans or were they goin' straight home?" Liz asked.

"Truth is, Granny, they were gonna go campin' for a few days." Mark answered.

"Son, you coulda gone with 'em, we wouldn't a minded." George interjected.

"Thanks, I guess I knew that, I just wanted to go home with you two, it'd give us some time to visit. If we're goin' on tour in the next couple a' months, I wanna spend as much time as possible with you both before I go."

Liz closed her eyes and said a brief, silent thank-you to her god.

"I'm glad you decided that Mark. We love having' you." Liz said as she grabbed his head and pulled it towards her for a kiss.

"Hey, Granny, I thought we were cuttin' down on kissin'?" He looked at Liz and gave her a happy grin.

It seemed like an eternity, the long drive home. Liz was quiet, thinking throughout most of the trip. She felt heaviness in her chest, and it wasn't her heart. At least not the doctor part. It's all the changes, she considered, Mark's comin' and goin', the girls, never coming home. It's just the changes.

As George turned onto their street, she realized she had been almost completely silent for the last two hours.

Home again, god I'm so glad! It's my favorite part of the trip, pullin' into my own driveway.

"What'ya thinkin' about, Sweetie?" George asked, walked into the house and pulled off their coats.

"I'm goin' downstairs and unpack right away. Gotta start practicin' for the next audition." Mark interrupted as he flew past them.

"That boy, will he never get enough of that music? Oh well, I'm glad that he's got a music addiction instead of another kind," said Liz.

"Yeah, wasn't Albert about his age when he got in that accident after a drinkin' party?"

"Sure was, George, we are blessed with Mark, aren't we?"

"Yes, Honey, we sure are."

"Let's make some coffee and see if there's anything to eat. I could use somethin'. How 'bout you?"

"Sure," Liz said.

They walked to the kitchen and Liz had a feast on the table in minutes.

"Lizzie, you are wonderful, but I didn't want you to go to all this trouble."

"mmmm,I did it because I'm as hungry as you are and glad to back in my own kitchen, making my own food."

"You didn't answer before. You were so quiet in the car, what'ya been thinkin' about?"

"Oh, George,, nothin' really, just gettin' use to all the changes around here. I mean the changes in my life."

"What changes, Sweetie, besides Mark's leaving'? Is there anything else?"

"No,, not really. Guess I'm just feelin' my age. I feel older than I have for a long time. When I look in the mirror, there's no changin' the fact that I'm seventy-ish."

"Are you sad? I think you look beautiful, wrinkles and all." George said as he motioned for Liz to sit on his lap. "Do you feel alright, Liz, I mean, physically?"

"Yeah, yeah, I'm fine. And, I went through the change years ago, so it's not that. I don't know exactly what it is, 'cept I'm just getting used to life the way it is now. Can't explain it any other way. I think," she added a little more brightly, "the best thing to do is just ignore me until this mood, or whatever passes."

"Is there anything I can do for you, Sweetie. I hate to see you like this."

"Like I said, best thing is just to ignore me. I do love a hug once in a while, though." Liz finished, laying her head on George's shoulder.

"Hey guys, should I come back later," Mark said as he breezed into the kitchen while George and Liz were embracing.

"You've caught us kissin' a few times in our life, no reason we should hide from you now." Liz said.

"A, few times?" Mark laughed.

"Alright, alright, young man, you never mind now and don't embarrass your Grandma." George said.

"I never worry about embarrassing Granny. You're much easier to embarrass than Granny is." Mark retorted.

All of them laughed at that. Liz knew that her mood couldn't hang on too long with these guys around.

****

"Mark, Mark!" Liz hollered as she saw the car pull into the driveway. "George, it's Mark, he's home! He's home!"

She opened the front door and ran to the approaching car. She saw Mark, in the back seat. <u>Oh, I've missed you so much, so much, my sweetie.</u>

"Granny!" He said as he climbed over another young man to get out of the car and throw his arms around her. "I missed you, Granny."

They were inside and talking in seconds. Liz, as always was putting food on the table. She had baked two peach pies for his homecoming. It seemed as if he had just come in from school, instead returning from a trip to Las Vegas.

"Well, Mark-o, did ya knock'em dead?" She asked him.

"Sure did, Granny sure did. We had a standing ovation every night. And....and, the big news, well..."

"Spit it out, boy, what's the big news? Wait let's get George in here. George, GEORGE," she hollered.

"Comin', cripes sakes, can't a guy even go to the john?" George hollered back as he came into the kitchen still zipping his pants.

"Well, Mark says there's big news and I didn't want to wait and I didn't want you to miss it, Old Man," she replied saucily. He sat in his chair at the head of the table and Liz sat down on his lap.

"Okay, c'mon, let's hear it," she remarked.

"Well, the fourth night we were there the manager of the place pulls me aside after our set. He asks me to come to his office. I'm a nervous wreck. I figure he's gonna can us and we won't get paid and the band'll split up and on and on. Anyways, I follow him into his office and there's another man waitin' for us."

"Who was it, c'mon, Mark, you're killin' us by draggin' this out," she said.

"Now, Grandmother, be patient." He said with a huge grin. "Let me see if I can remember," he added just to prolong her torture.

She reached across the table and gave him her gentle mother-bear swat to the head, "Now quit foolin' around and tell us what went on!"

Mark smiled at Liz. <u>Nineteen and he still looks like an angel,</u> she thought as he continued his story.

"Well...we, the band and I, we got a TOUR!"

Liz looked at George, then at Mark, "A what, you got a what?"

"A tour, Granny, the big time, I mean we're not the headliners for the tour, we're the lead-in act for the Screamin Apes.

"You mean that band you sang first for in Las Vegas the first time?," Liz asked.

"Yup, they're the biggest right now and they liked our act so much they want us to go on tour with them and open all their shows. That was the other man in the office, the manager for the Apes. Can you believe it? Granny, how will I ever repay you for all you've done for me? You've always been there for me, loved me, taken care of me and now, you are the one who, single-handedly, got my career goin. All my success is because of you. Hell, all I am is because of you!" Mark finished quietly.

Liz noticed tears in Mark's eyes. It was the first time she had seen him cry since he was a little boy. She rose from her chair and went to him. They hugged long and hard. Liz softly patted Mark's back during the entire embrace. <u>I wish I</u>

<u>could keep him this close forever. It's almost as if he were small again, needing a good, strong mother-hug. I wish I could always be there when he needed one.</u>

"Granny," Mark said, breaking the silence, "I want to do something really special for you."

"Don't forget to thank George, honey, he's done as much or more for you than I have," she interrupted.

"Oh, no I haven't," George piped in, "We all know who has been the most important person to Mark. I've been happy to play the part in his life that I have, but it's nowhere near the energy, work, or caring that you've contributed."

"Oh, George...oh, Mark," was all she could say, she knew her lip was quivering more than it ever had.

"No cryin' now Granny, this is the best time. I'm gonna, somehow, make you happy!" Mark said. Then he laughed and hugged Liz another time.

"I've never been as happy as I am right now!" She said quietly, wiping tears from her cheeks.

"I know you hate it when I'm gone , but I will call all the time and I'm gonna send you guys tickets to come to some of the cities I'll be playin' in. It could be like mini-vacations. You could have lots of second honeymoons and I'd make sure you're treated like royalty. Remember you're the parents of a star, now. You gotta get used to it."

"This is so wonderful, Mark, we're so proud of you. You've come so far and it's been only a year since graduation. Take your fame slowly, though, son, learn to use it wisely." George said.

Chapter Eleven

Liz knew she had to call Mark soon, let him know the news. First, she had to tell George.

How am I going to do it? How do I tell the man I love that my time is coming to an end. I don't want to leave him. I don't want to leave this world, but I refuse to be a burden and I know George will insist on keeping me alive long past the time I should be. She was still too shocked to cry. The doctor told her this morning. He wanted to schedule surgery as soon as possible. This will ruin Mark's tour, she thought. Why did it have to happen? I'm not ready to die. What'd he say? I asked him what kind of chance I had of beating this. Oh, yeah, he said, "we'll see," sounds real hopeful.

Liz pulled in the drive and walked slowly into the house. She felt as if she were walking through mud. It was like a dream where you can't run away from the monsters no matter how hard you try. Liz felt the monster inside her and knew it would eventually engulf her.

"Hi, Sweetie," George called from the kitchen as she opened the front door.

"Hi," she called back. I don't want to tell him. God make something happen so I don't have to look at him when I tell him. Please let me die right now so I don't have to see him suffer.

No luck, no lightening, nothing', guess I got to face him.

She walked to the kitchen. George greeted her with a huge bear hug.

"How's my love, today?" He asked.

"Oh, I'm okay," she said quietly.

"You, sure,, Sweetie? I don't see your usual big smile."

"Might as well get to it," she said, almost in a whisper, "I guess I'm not quite as right as I'd like to be, George."

"Well, tell me about it. What's wrong?"

She gritted her teeth. She could already see the panic in his face.

"George, hold my hand, will ya?"

"Sure, Sweetie, what's wrong? Just tell me, you know it always helps when we talk."

"It won't help this time, I'm afraid. I went to the doctor, George, ya know, just for a check-up."

"Uh-huh...He found somethin', didn't he?"

"Yes, George,, a ...a tumor, a tumor on my left lung."

Saying it like that, out loud, with George listening to every word, made it terribly real. She was going to die, soon. She was going to leave her family and have to suffer horribly before the monster would finally kill her. What had she ever done to deserve this? Why did it happen? Where was God, now? She knew her lip was past quivering. She felt warm tears rolling down her face.

In a moment she was in George's arms. He lifted her and sat her on his lap, his strong arms surrounding her. She buried her face in his shoulder and let herself sob.

Liz finally raised her head from George's shoulder to notice the sun dipping below the horizon. She faced the kitchen window and the west, as the sun disappeared, bright rays of pink and orange and red shot skyward. <u>Like me, the sun is dying. I guess that's what my life has been, those rays of red and orange before the darkness. I guess it's time to face the night.</u>

"When do you think we should let the kids know?" George asked a few minutes later.

"The kids...oh, you mean LeeAnn, Lisa, and Albert?"

"And,... Mark," George added.

"Mark, oh...God, Mark, I've got to tell Mark!" Liz began to cry again. "Isn't enough that I have this thing and I'm going to die from it. Why do I have to torture my family and watch their pain?" She asked.

"Lizzie, Sweetie, I will not hear any more talk of death. We're gonna see you through this thing and have lots of years to go. It'll be hard on you, girl, I know, but don't give up so soon." He took her face in his hands and looked into her eyes, "You are going to make it, my love, I guarantee it and you know I don't believe in lying. Do you believe me; will you work hard to beat this?"

"Yes,, you old thing. I believe you. I'll try hard to live," she said while thinking, I'm <u>sorry, my love, I know when I'm beat. I know I won't make it, but I'll keep trying for you, only for you and Mark.</u>

They talked and decided to call Mark that evening. Liz knew she had to be the one to break the news and she wanted to tell him before he came home. She didn't want him hysterically trying to get home to find out what was wrong.

"How 'bout if I fix us some supper, Sweetie?" George asked.

"I'm not dead yet!" Liz remarked smartly, "there'll be plenty of time for you to learn how to cook later, for now I'm the main cook in this family."

"Honey, don't ever forget how much I love you," George said as Liz rose from his lap.

"I know, George, I always knew it and I always will."

Liz started to look through the cupboards and the refrigerator while she talked. "How 'bout some pork chops and scalloped potatoes, sounds good on a cold fall night, doesn't it?"

"Sure does, you sure you're up to it?"

"I gotta do somethin', George or I'm gonna explode with anger or bein' afraid, or... or... I don't know what." Liz answered as she started peeling potatoes.

"Okay, I think I understand. I'm glad you still wanna cook, seems somehow more normal, as if all this wasn't real."

"I wish it wasn't real, but wishin' doesn't make anything real, does it?"

"No, Sweetie, but prayin' does." George answered.

Liz looked at him, but made no comment. She knew she wasn't sure enough that prayer might save her. She hoped George's faith would work its magic for her.

A few moments later, George told her he'd call the three oldest.

"I just don't know how to say it to them, George, and if they were angry with me or thinkin' I wanted them to take care of me or somethin'. I don't know how I'd feel. It would be better if you called."

George nodded a silent agreement, rose from his seat, and walked into the dining room to make the call.

Liz continued her preparations, working furiously and noisily, she did not want to hear what George was saying to the kids.

"Well, they all took it real well, Liz." George said after the call.

"Did anyone complain that I'd be too much to take care of?" Liz asked, expecting at least one of them to say something along those lines.

"No, no one made mention of anything like that. All of them just said they were real worried about you and that they wanted to be here when you had surgery."

"That figures, now that I'm dying, they'll come see me. It would be the first time since Mark came to live with us that Lisa or Lee Ann came. I somehow can't imagine what it would be like, to have them here. Too bad I had to get cancer before they'd come. Maybe I shoulda done it a long time ago."

"Sweetie," George said quietly, "You have every reason in the world to be bitter and angry with the kids, but don't waste the good time that you've got on anger, okay? I think it might just give that tumor the kind of body it wants to grow in. Cancer must be evil; it needs anger and evil or it will grow. Don't feed it, okay?"

"George you never stop amazin' me, ya know." Liz said as she left supper preparations to give her husband a huge hug. She clung to him for a minute and whispered, "I'll do anything it takes to stay with you as long as possible."

<u>I've just committed myself to face this thing and fight hard. Oh, God give me strength to beat it. I do want to live. I want to be with my George for a lot longer. Give me the strength to fight.</u>

Liz enjoyed the quiet supper with George. Mark had been away for several months; they had had many suppers alone. This one, though, was different. She couldn't remember she felt so close to George. <u>It's almost as if the monster didn't exist, at least not for right now.</u>

Liz knew they'd have to call Mark that evening. She wanted him home for the surgery, but she would never ask him directly. <u>He has too much goin' on in his life right now. I'm not going' to drag him away from his first tour just to sit in some waiting room while I'm unconscious. I hope he wants to come when the tour takes a break. I think around the holidays they have a couple of days without shows.</u> She would encourage him to come then.

She held the receiver in her hand for a long time before dialing. George had placed a kitchen chair near their old phone table so that she could sit and talk as long as necessary.

"George, I'm not sick yet, you old fuss bug!" she scolded him as he brought the chair to her.

"Yeah, yeah, I know, but I also know you and you're gonna want to talk a long time. Might as well be comfortable." He then winked and kissed her on the cheek.

She could feel her lip quivering already and knew that she'd better get the words out, tell Mark, before her voice failed completely.

"Hi, Granny, is that you, Sweetie? ...can hardly hear you with all the noise from the bands, let me call you back from my room. It'll take only a couple'a minutes to get up there. I'll be right back."

George poked his face through the kitchen door.

"What's up, Sweetie? You hung up so fast."

"I had Mark paged when he didn't answer his room phone. I must'a caught him between acts or somethin'. He couldn't hear over all the noise in the lounge, so he said he'd call....there he is,"

She interrupted herself as the phone rang.

George disappeared into the kitchen. Liz was alone to give her Mark-o the news.

"That's better, Granny, now I don't hafta yell everything, either. What's up? How are you and George? Gee, I miss you both so much. We get standing ovations every time we're on stage, can you believe it?"

"Oh, I can believe it. I know how good you are. You sound pretty excited, have you had a good time, Mark? Is the tour fun?"

"Oh, gosh, Granny, it's the best thing in the world. I can't believe we actually make money doing something that's so much fun as this."

"I'm so glad for you, my love..." she said, wondering if it was time to let him know.

"How 'bout you guys? How are you doin'? Is everything all right?"

"Well, Mark-o, that's why I called. I have some kinda bad news, but not horrible, I mean we don't even know, yet, what it means."

"What is it, Granny?" Mark asked. Liz noticed he didn't sound as happy as he had at first.

"Well, son, I've got to have some surgery next week. The doctor saw a shadow on my left lung, on a routine x-ray and he thinks I should have it taken care of right away."

There was silence for a moment or two. Liz did not want to intrude into that time. It was the time Mark needed to absorb what she said.

"Granny..." he said tentatively, at last, "what day is your surgery, I'll be home for it or before, if I can get a flight."

"Now, now, Mark-o, don't you think it's kinda silly for you to come and watch me sleep. Take your time. Come a few days after, when I'm not so uncomfortable and will be awake more. There's no need for you to rush."

"That's ridiculous!" Mark answered with an angry edge to his voice, "Are you saying you don't want me, 'cuz in that case I won't come."

"Oh, Mark-o, you know I don't mean that for a minute," She could feel her lip starting its dance. "I want you here, honest, more than anything. I just didn't think it was right to make you come to my side for this stupid old shadow thing." She could feel the tears building behind the dam of her lower lids.

"Stupid, Granny, it's not a stupid thing, it's serious and I love you. Do you think I would ever want to miss being close to you when you'll be needing as much love and caring as we can give? This is the kind of time, you and George taught me, that families stick together. I'll be there, what day did you say?"

She gave him the times and date of her tests, ten a.m. next Tuesday. "They'll decide if and when the surgery will be depending on the tests," she said. She loved hearing his voice; its strength gave her strength. <u>Another reason to live, I want to see Mark's success, or failure. I want to be part of his life for a long time.</u>

"Thanks for telling me, Granny, I want to be there for everything, you should know that. I'll come in on Monday night so get the pinochle cards warmed up," he said to end the conversation.

■■■

<u>He's here. I can relax, my Mark-o's home. I know everything will work out now. My Mark-o's home.</u>

Liz hugged Mark long and hard the minute he walked in the front door. She had been cooking all day, making pies, a huge roast, and a multitude of side dishes. The smell of all that home cooking filled every corner of the house.

"Geez, Granny, you musta been on a real cookin' binge, huh," Mark said as he smiled at her and removed his coat. "I think I could smell this as we flew over on the way to the airport." He teased.

She couldn't stop looking at him; her hand remained on his shoulder as they started for the kitchen. George, who had picked up Mark at the airport, followed behind them.

"Hey, Sweetie, don't I get that kind of a hug, too," George said in mock jealously.

"Oh, you, didn't we do enough of that all night?" Liz answered with glance and a grin directed at her husband. Their night long antics would be a treasured memory through the long weeks of surgery and recuperation. She noticed George smiled widely in return.

"Guess you two have been as close as ever," Mark interjected.

"Never you mind, you're too young to know about such things. Besides, nothing wrong with an old married couple cavort in' in the way God intended for married couples, is there?" Liz asked.

"Absolutely nothing' wrong with it. In fact I'm awful glad to know you guys are still engaged in such things," Mark answered.

"Well, shadow or no, I'm not dead yet and I'm plannin' lots more nights like last night after all this nonsense is over." Liz said.

They ate and talked all evening, it was after eight when Mark offered to clear the table and set up the cards for their night's entertainment.

Liz noticed that their card game was much quieter than usual. <u>It's me, she thought, I'm usually the one that makes the most noise. Just can't tonight, not quite up to it. I like to be with them though; just sittin' here with them is enough for tonight.</u>

"It was a good night, old man," she said as she climbed into bed after midnight.

"It's so good to have him home. I'm so glad he wanted to come. It's good to have you here, too, of course. I couldn't do this, wouldn't want to, without you guys."

George put his arms around her. They were as close as possible in the big old double bed they had shared since their marriage. Liz had been afraid she would never be able to sleep, but the busy day and Mark's arrival had worn her out. She was warm and felt safe in George's arms. She felt herself floating off into sleep. Her last thought was one of sadness, somehow she felt this was the last time she'd be so peaceful.

Liz was awake before the alarm went off at six. She was not supposed to eat anything or drink anything except clear liquids since midnight of the night before her test. <u>They'll never be able to tell and I wouldn't be able to live without my coffee. You can't tell me that a coupl'a cups of black coffee will hurt anything.</u> As soon as the brewing stopped, she poured herself a large cup of the rich liquid and sat in her favorite chair. After the first sip, she was sure she could stand just about anything. <u>That's better!</u>

"Good morning, bright eyes," George said as he joined her.

He looked at the cup as she raised it to her lips.

"Don't you say a thing," she warned.

"Who,, me? Never in a million years." He answered.

Mark greeted them with a sleepy, "Mornin'," just as they were putting on their coats.

"Thought you'd oversleep and miss goin' with us," Liz said.

"No chance, I'm just not used to this early stuff. Life on the road means going to bed at three a.m., not gettin' up 'til one or two in the afternoon, at the earliest!"

"Do you want us to wait a few minutes to let you get ready?" She asked.

"I'm all ready," he answered as he kissed her cheek and grabbed his own coat. "Let's go."

****

"Whoever thought up those god-awful ways of torturin' people, I'd like to meet and make sure they got some of their own medicine." Were the first words out of Liz' mouth as she exited radiology and met George and Mark.

"That bad,, huh, Sweetie?" George asked.

"Worse!" Was all she'd say?

"I bet you'd feel a lot better with some food in your stomach, let's get a bite at the coffee shop. Bet a big ol' piece a pie and a hot cuppa coffee will fix you right up." Mark offered.

Liz looked at him and smiled a little, <u>he always knows how to make me feel better.</u>

"Now we just gotta wait, I guess." Liz said after finishing her pie and coffee.

"Did they say how long ya gotta wait before they decide what's goin' on?" George asked.

"They just said Dr. Black would call after he and the radiologist looked over all the tests. Maybe it'll take'em till Christmas, so I don't havta have anything done 'til then."

"Liz, that'd be over two months from now, I kinda doubt it."

"Besides, Granny," Mark piped in, "You're gonna be well long before Christmas. Like George said, that's over two months from now. I know nothing will keep you down that long!"

****

Liz was alone, sipping coffee and casually reading the paper. She struggled, since the day of the tests, to hide her constant state of anxiety. She was on edge every moment. She knew she jumped at any sudden noise, cried whenever she was alone and never slept. She did not want George or Mark to worry about her, so she did her best to hide the signs of her nervousness

She glanced at the kitchen clock, eight a.m. and all's well, so far. I know they're gonna call today.

It was Friday, three days since her tests and plenty of time for the doctors to read whatever it was they read to determine her fate. She knew in her heart what those tests would show, she had known for quite a while, something was wrong. She had blamed her ill feelings on Mark's leaving, on age, on some flu bug, on anything but what her heart told her from the beginning. Her body was beginning to die.

The phone rang a little before ten. Liz was washing breakfast dishes when she heard George answer it.

"Hello, yes, this is the Ostlund's. Just a second and I'll get her. Honey, it's for you, the doctor.

Liz felt her heart beating hard and fast. She wiped her hands on a towel and walked, slowly to the phone. She smiled at George and patted his hand as she took the receiver, "It'll be okay, you'll see."

"Hello, Dr. Black, yes this is Liz. You have news for me?"

"Yes, Liz and I'm afraid it's not especially good news. Why don't you come into the office for a talk? I'd like to discuss all your options and it would be much better, for you, if we did that here at my office."

Her knees felt weak, she sat down still holding the receiver, her lip quivering. "I need to know right now, Doctor. What did you find? I can't come into the office today. I need to be here with my family and you can talk about options just as well over this damn thing as you could if I drove the two hours to see you."

Dr. Black seemed to be hesitating. The phone was quiet for hours, it seemed. "Dr. Black, please tell me now."

"Liz, this is against my better judgment,, but, okay, have it your way. You probably will want to be close to your family. Is George still there?"

"Standing right beside me." As she said it, she grabbed George's hand and squeezed it tightly.

"Well, Liz,, that spot on your lung is not your big problem. You have a large, very invasive tumor of your kidney. We feel that the malignancy there has spread to your lung and we need to remove both tumors as soon as possible."

She let out a tiny breath of air with an almost imperceptible squeak. She felt as if she were in a dream and trying to scream but couldn't. Large...malignancy...tumors, God, God, God....

"Liz, honey...Liz, let me have the phone."

A male voice, she wasn't sure who's, told her to relinquish the thing in her hand. She did that as the horrible words continued racing through her brain. Was that George next to her? <u>Why in God's green earth is he talking on the phone? Doesn't he know I'm dying.</u>

****

Liz was vaguely aware that someone had entered the room.

"Liz, honey, Liz, try to wake up, honey, I'm so worried about you."

It was George speaking to her. "What's a matter, Love, time to get up? Did I oversleep?" She asked, thinking it might be morning and she was supposed to be somewhere.

"No, Sweetie, you kinda fainted an hour ago. I brought you in here to rest. How do you feel? Are you any better?"

She remembered. She had a malignancy, that's what the doctor had said. It wasn't morning. It was afternoon and she was going to die real soon. She had cancer.

"George, hold me will you. I'm so cold." She said.

"Don't you worry, Sweetie, I'll hold you always and forever. I'll never let you go. Don't you worry, we'll get through this, you and I and Mark. We'll get through this together."

"Oh, god, I've got to tell Mark! Oh, George, please don't make me tell him! I can't say the words. I don't want him to see how scared I am. Will you tell him?"

"Already did, Sweetie. Had to. I needed his help to get you out of the chair and into bed. He's a smart boy. He had it figured out before I opened my mouth. He loves you so much, Liz, it's almost as hard on him as it is on you. Can I let him in to see you? He's dyin' to."

She felt as if the wind had been knocked out of her. She was finally catching her breath. She wasn't going to let the old, spit-in-your-eye, fightin' Liz disappear now. She needed her strength and her cynicism, if she had any chance at all to beat this. "Give me a minute to quit this weepin' crap, and then I wanna see him too! God, I can't believe I lost it like that. I've never, under any circumstances, let anything hit me like this has, but I'm over it and now I'll start fightin'. Got too much left to do, before I let some god-awful disease kill Me., Right?" She said as she looked, again, into her husband's eyes.

He had been crying too. It was the first time Liz could ever remember seeing George cry. She reached up and wiped the tears from his cheeks, then kissed him long and hard. "I am NOT dead yet, right!" She said firmly.

"Sure as hell not," he answered.

"Then I gotta get my strength together for the fight, don't I?"

"Yup."

"We can do it. I'll come through it, I know. When's the surgery?" she asked George.

"Doctor Black scheduled you for Tuesday morning. They'll do the kidney first and a week later, take out that spot on your lung, if you're up for it."

"Have you ever known me not to be up to something?" She asked suddenly feeling as irreverent as always.

George laughed, "God, Lizzie, you're the only woman I know who could come up with a line like that one after hearin' what you heard today. I do expect you'll get through this. You're just too ornery and stubborn to let anything, even a disease overpower you."

Chapter Twelve

"Granny, are you scared?" Mark asked.

She had to admit that she was, but only to herself. If she said the words out loud, God might hear them. She was determined that no one but George would ever know her fears.

"Honey, I'm not scared one bit. These doctors do this stuff all the time; didn't you know your granny's invincible?" Liz was lying on a surgical cart; George and Mark were leaning over the side rails, holding her hands and patting her face. "You two look like nervous Nellies hangin' over a crib for god sakes. I'll be more than fine. Wooo, that shot they gave me; I'm startin' to feel like I've had three martinis. This could be fun."

George looked down at her and smiled. Mark simply stood there patting her hand. I wish they'd just let me go to sleep and get this over with. I'm sure tired of worryin' about it.

"Mrs. Ostlund, Elizabeth Ostlund," she heard someone say.

"Over here, I'm the one havin' the party," she hollered in response.

"Well, dear," a woman in green clothes and a paper hat on hung over the railing of her cart, "I'm Ms. Stewart, your nurse. We're ready for you in surgery."

"Guess I gotta go, guys. Listen, I...I love you both so much," was all she could say. Oh, god, I'm gonna cry, can't do that. I'll just keep my lips tight and no one'll know.

"Love you, Granny," Mark said as he leaned farther over the rail to kiss her forehead. "We'll be right with you when you wake up. I love you."

She looked at him, tried to smile to reassure him. She knew, though, if she relaxed for an instant, to speak or smile, the tears would flow. I don't want him rememberin' me that way.

"Love you, Sweetie, more than I can say." George whispered as he kissed her. "Behave yourself and don't give those doctors any problems, okay?"

She nodded. The cart started moving. The tears came. <u>Guess this is it.</u>

****

"Remember that first surgery?" I asked George. We were in the waiting room for the thousandth time. It's been a week since we learned Liz was not ever coming home. She seemed weaker every day. For the last twenty-four hours she had been slipping in and out of consciousness. The nurses and doctors came in frequently to change this dressing or that, or to regulate one of the multitudes of machines that whirred and buzzed around her. We found ourselves in the waiting room frequently. I guess they chased us out to "spare us" from seeing her suffer. They didn't know that nothing could spare us; we were hurting with her and for her, every minute of every day.

"God, yes, Mark, as if it were yesterday. We thought she'd do so well. She never gave up, Mark, you know that don't you? Even now, she's not given up."

"I know, George," I said putting my arm around his shoulder.

"I've been thinking, Mark, about that, ya know. I've been thinking about just that."

"What do you mean, George?" I asked him, knowing and refusing to know what he meant at the same time.

"Mark, Liz will keep on fighting for as long as her poor body holds out. Mark, don't you think she's fought enough? You know how much I love her, God, she's my life; but, she's been in terrible pain for six months, now. All she really wants is to go home, and I don't mean to the little house I built."

I couldn't imagine George ever saying anything like this, but I knew he was right. Liz was just holding on for me. She knew George would be alright. He'd be joining her soon. She was my mother and didn't want to leave me. She was still trying to prove to I-don't-know-who that she was a good mother and would never leave her child.

I looked at George and nodded, "I've got to be the one to tell her it's okay to go, don't I? I've got to be the one to tell her that her duty's been done and that she's been a wonderful mother. It's time for her to rest. I know, George, I will."

I knew at that moment the one way I could accomplish this awful task. I wanted her to know how much she meant to me all those years. She was my life. She taught me how to live and how to love. I had always had a nagging feeling that I needed to thank her in a way that was truly special, a way that reflected how special she had been to me. I had been working towards this all of my life. I had been working on a way to use the gifts I had to tell the world, and her, how the love she planted and nurtured in me had grown and made me what I am.

****

"Liz, Liz, honey, it's George and Mark," she heard the voice through the fog and darkness. <u>Where the hell am I? Can't remember, if it's night or day. What day is it? God, I'm tired. Why can't they leave me sleep?</u>

"Mrs. Ostlund, Liz, time to open your eyes. You've been sleeping a long time. We need to take your vital signs." Another voice, this was more persistent.

"Who are this damn we? ... Why the hell do I have to wake up if I don't want to?" Liz mumbled.

"C'mon Granny, we wanna see those gorgeous eye." This was Mark's voice and for that she managed to open her eyes just enough to see she wasn't at home. <u>The operation's over, I know now. I'm in the hospital. Still don't know why I gotta wake</u>

up.

She began to feel the pain in her left side, yup, operation's over, now I gotta put up with this.

"Are you hurting, Granny?" Mark's voice said.

Liz managed to nod and say, "What the hell do you think, I just had an operation!"

She heard George's voice say, "She's okay; whenever she's this grouchy you know everything's workin' the way it should."

Liz noticed the nurse enter the room and within seconds a wave of relief from the pain swept over her. Need to sleep a little more. Let me rest just a few more minutes.

The next few days in the hospital were not as hard, or as painful, as Liz had expected. She was out of bed and walking the halls by the second day and hollering for the doctor to release her on Friday.

"Please call my doctor, Dr. Black, and tell him I want outta here today," she shouted into her intercom at eight o'clock Friday morning.

"Doctor will be making rounds soon, Mrs. Ostlund," the voice from the wall answered, "We'll make sure he sees you first."

"Are you ready for me at home?" She asked George, who had been at the hospital since six at her insistence.

"Sure am, Honey, that's why I came in so early today. Can't wait to have you home."

"We gotta find out what the tests showed on that kidney before I leave, and then we gotta stop for groceries on the way home. I've gotta get a few things made up for you guys for the next time I'm in the hospital. I've been thinkin' about it and I don't think I left you enough frozen stuff to get you through the next few weeks."

"I'm sure there's plenty, Liz." George laughed and said, "The basement freezer's so full I can't open the door without bein' hit by a avalanche of frozen stuff. Besides, you don't think for one moment that we're gonna let you cook when you get home, do ya? Lizzie, you had one major surgery two days ago and got another one next week, for crissakes, you're gonna behave yourself."

It was the first time she had ever heard George be so forceful, "Guess you're right, Honey," she said, "I'm just feelin' so good and I'm so anxious to have life get back to normal. Maybe I am in a little too much of a hurry."

"Damn right you are! You're gonna go home and get pampered. We already got a hospital bed in the dining room so you don't have to do anything but lay there and be the center of everything. Promise me Liz."

"I promise, Sweetie." It'll be so good to get home, I'll promise anything.

****

Liz turned her face towards the car window. George was driving and Mark was in the back seat. No one had spoken since they left home. Liz could not look at her husband or at Mark; she could not stop her silent tears and did not want them to see her so upset. It was Tuesday; they were on the way to the hospital for the second surgery.

She managed to hide her tears, wiping away their stain before George parked. He put his arm around her to help her into the hospital. She had her arms around his waist. She hugged tightly and let go very reluctantly when they reached the admission area.

"Granny, I love you so much." Mark said, "It'll be over fast, you'll see, just like last week and you'll be home again for the weekend."

"I know, sweetie, I'll be fine as soon as we get this goin'. The hard part is this waitin' and gettin' ready, ya know what I mean?" Mark nodded in response.

A nurse walked over to them and said, "Time to go and get ready. We'll get you back with your family after you're prepped."

Liz grabbed George and kissed him. "Love ya," she said quickly.

She kissed Mark on the cheek and walked away with the nurse.

****

Where were Mark and George? Why would no one answer when she called? Liz had been in this dark place for what seemed like days. There were no lights, no sound, only hot, searing pain and short movie-like scenes of her and Mark and George years ago. She'd see herself caring for Mark as a baby, rushing him to the hospital when he took the pills, watching his Little League game, then the blackness would come again. Where was she? Was this heaven or hell? <u>Got to get outta here, but too tired. Rest a little, and then try to get up. If I can move, maybe I'll wake up or not. Wonder if I'm dead or alive. So tired now,, though. Need to rest again.</u>

"Granny, please wake up, we miss you." She heard Mark's voice. It was strong and it sounded as if he was right next to her.

She tried again to move. <u>Open those eyelids, girl, what the hell is the matter with you? C'mon body, move, work, just the eyelids, that's it! That's it, I can see! I'm alive, that's Mark right there. Maybe...I'll try. Yes! I can move my fingers! He took my hand! George, it's George, too. Oh, God, I'm alive, thank-you.</u>

"Granny, you're awake!" Mark practically screamed.

George was standing on the other side of the bed. She looked up at him and saw him smiling from ear to ear. It was so difficult to speak, but she wanted them to know she was okay.

"I'm okay," she said very quietly. "I came back didn't I?"

George nodded and lifted her hand to his lips. He kissed her fingers.

"Granny, we missed you so." Mark said. He was holding her other hand.

"I know, sweetie, I missed you guys, too!" She said it and felt herself drifting away. <u>It's okay. I'm just going to sleep. So tired,, again. But I'm okay. I'm back.</u>

Liz wakened again. "What the hell time is it anyway? How long have I been out of surgery?" She asked. She didn't see anyone standing by her bed; she assumed that there was someone close by.

"Granny?" Mark questioned as he suddenly appeared at her side.

<u>He looks worn out,</u> she thought. "It's me, Mark-o, what time is it? Seems like, I've been out for a while."

"You sure have, it's Friday, Granny."

"Oh my god, I've been out for more than three days?" <u>No wonder I thought I was dead.</u> "What happened, why did I sleep so long?"

"Dr. Black said the surgery went fine, you were just a little more worn out than he figured. He said you were fightin' to wake up though. We were awful worried."

"Where's George?" she asked.

"He's down getting some breakfast in the cafeteria. I fell asleep in the chair. We both stayed here all night and all day since the operation."

"Mark, is she awake? Did I hear you talkin' to Liz?" George boomed as he walked into the room.

"She's awake!" Mark shouted excitedly.

"Hi, sweetie," George said very quietly as he came to her side, took her hand, and kissed it. "We were wonderin' when you'd come back to us."

"I really didn't want to be away, honest," Liz looked at her husband and felt a warm flush of love for him. "I love you so much, the two of you!"

"Now you're back and we're gonna get you strong enough to get home, soon as possible, okay?" Mark said.

"Fine with me," Liz answered.

****

Liz tried as hard as she could every day. She tried to do the strengthening exercises with the physical therapist. She tried to do the breathing exercises with the respiratory therapist and she tried to eat the food that was served to her.

"If you don't eat, you won't ever get out of here," the nurse had told her this morning; but, in the two weeks following the surgery she couldn't do it. At first she'd throw up every time she tried. After days of vomiting, she simply stopped trying.

"The doctor has given you enough medicine to calm your stomach down, now it's up to you to eat." That same nurse said at lunch time.

<u>Something's wrong and I can't tell what it is or how to stop it. Everything's gettin' worse, no matter how much I fight this thing. I know somethin' is horribly wrong. I don't think I'll ever get outta this, but I promised my Mark-o and I gotta keep tryin'.</u>

George and Mark were there, by her side, all day, and every day. She knew she was disappointing them by not getting well. She could see it in their faces.

<u>God, I feel cold,</u> she considered as her lunch tray was taken away. <u>I'm hot one minute and cold the next. My chest hurts and I'm freezing, but I don't want to let on about it. I must seem like the biggest cry baby in the whole world, all I do is complain about how bad I feel. Gotta stop it. Gotta just fight and keep my aches and pains to myself. George and Mark gotta get some rest and I can't disappoint them.</u>

"Why don't you guys go on home for the afternoon? I'm gonna nap and try to get feelin' a little better. Go on now, get your butts outa here and leave me rest alone! Why don't you bring me a hamburger and some fries for dinner? It sounds kinda good." She said while curling up in bed as if she were going to sleep.

<u>That'll fool'em. They'll do anything to get me to eat, including leaving for</u>

awhile. When they leave I can get the nurse to get me a pain shot and not have them worryin' about it.

"You sure,, Granny?" Mark asked.

"Honey, you've been so sweet to me. Did I ever even thank you for gettin' the kids to say they were sorry? You're the one who got them here and made them feel so guilty they were fallin' all over themselves with apologies. It's good I made things better between us, Mark and you're the ones who did it. You've done so much, honey and because of it I know I'm gettin' better, honest. Now, I don't want you gettin' sick, just when I'm plannin' on bein' well."

She pulled Mark down to her and kissed his cheek, then whispered, "Get George home and get him some rest."

"No problem," Mark whispered back. Then said aloud, "Let's go, George, Liz's got the right idea. We all need a break, her included."

George kissed her and touched her cheek. He seemed reluctant but promised her he'd rest up.

When they left, Liz called for the nurse. The pain in her chest had grown to crushing proportions. Her breath came in short, sharp bursts.

"Can I help you?" The voice in the wall asked.

"Please, help, I...I can't ...breathe." Liz managed to stammer.

"We're on our way!" Liz heard.

Hold on, girl, calm down, breathe, help's coming. She said to herself again and again, until she saw a woman come into the room. The room darkened, she realized her vision was failing. The last thing she heard was a loud voice screaming, Code Blue Room 304.

Liz was aware of George and Mark coming and going. She'd awaken and they'd be there. Another time she woke to find a stranger doing strange things to the various tubes that seemed to be sprouting from every spot on her body.

At times she knew that she was in the hospital and moving between her dreams and wakefulness. At other times she was lost, confused and wondering where she was and why so many people seemed so intent on hurting her.

Chapter Thirteen

"George, do you think she hears me? Do you think she knows what I'm saying? It's been what, .a week now. I've been tellin' her it's okay to go, to leave. I don't know if she even hears me." I said as George and I sat drinking our millionth cup of hospital coffee.

"Mark, she doesn't respond to anyone. I have to believe she understands, though. She's never been this peaceful. The last few times she went into this coma-thing, she was restless and like fightin' every minute. Remember how they had to give her medicine to quiet her, even when she wasn't really awake?"

"Yup."

"Son, you're doin' the right thing. God knows I'm not brave enough to tell her it's okay to die. Damn it! I want her around. I wanna be the one to go first. I don't wanna be alone. Now if that ain't the most selfish thing you ever heard." George said and looked at me. His eyes were close to overflowing with the tears I knew he was always trying to hold back.

"George," I said as I reached for his hand across the cafeteria table, "I won't ever let you be alone, not ever."

He nodded then got up from his chair, "Guess we better get back there, I don't wanna have her alone whenever the time does come.

We made the trek back to her room. The halls were so familiar to me that I never even thought about how to get there, I think my feet knew the way on their own. I wonder how many times, in the last six months I had walked this same path.

"Mr. Ostlund, Mr. Ostlund," one of the nurses said loudly as we approached the station, "We were just going to page you, I think you'd better go in to your wife."

George and I looked at each other. Everyone knows what that statement means. My heart dropped to my stomach. I could hear the sudden "thunk" as it hit bottom. Today, April 28, would be Liz Ostlund's last day on earth and the end of all life as I had known it.

"Liz, honey, Mark and I are here with you." George said gently as he took her hand.

I joined him, at her bedside, and took her other hand. There were so many things I wanted to say. Damn it, she might not even hear me! It didn't matter; I had to tell her how I felt.

"Granny, my love, I know you're leavin' us now. It's my own fault, I guess, 'cuz I told you it was okay to go. It is, you need your rest and release from your pain, but it isn't okay 'cuz I don't know how I'll live without you."

I sat in a chair at her bedside and laid my head on her pillow, "I'll miss you always, dear lady. I'll never let a day go by when I don't think of you and all you've done for me. You've taught me everything about love, honor, respect, honesty and truthfulness. Memories of your lessons and your love will keep me going; will keep me close to you, always.

Your love kept me warm on the coldest days, your smile made even the darkest days, bright." I kissed her and noticed her breathing had slowed, the time was close.

"Before you leave us I have one small gift to give you. I've been working on it for years and waiting for the perfect time to give it to you. I may have waited too long. I just hope you can hear this and know how much you have meant to me."

Now, was the time to give her the gift I had slaved over for so many years? I had tried to give it to her many times in the past, but never felt it was the right time. Then, before I had the chance, she was comatose and I figured, unable to receive it. I want to give it to her anyway. I want to sing the song I wrote for her and hope she hears it before she dies.

"Sweetie," I whispered to her, "I hope you hear this, I wrote this song for you." I started to sing softly, close to her ear:

MY GRANNY, I ALWAYS LOVED BEING YOUR SON
FROM THE DAY I FIRST KNEW YOU, YOU WERE ALWAYS THE ONE
WHEN I CRIED, YOU WERE THERE WITH A REASSURING HUG
MY DEAR GRANNY, YOU'RE A SPECIAL LADY IN EACH AND EVERY WAY
MY LOVE AND ADMIRATION FOR YOU GREW MORE AND MORE EACH DAY
YOU ALWAYS ALLOWED ME TO BE ME. YOU TAUGHT ME THE WAY
TO SHOW OTHERS I CARE, TO LAUGH AND TO LOVE AND HOW ALL OF US MUST SHARE.
YOU NURTURED ME AND HELPED MAKE ALL MY DREAMS COME TRUE.
WHEN YOU'RE GONE, I'LL BE LOST. I CAN'T IMAGINE LIFE WITHOUT YOU.

MY DEAR GRANNY, YOU'RE A SPECIAL LADY IN EACH AND EVERY WAY,
AS A YOUNGSTER, I KNEW THIS AND THOSE FEELINGS GREW EACH DAY

DARLING GRANNY, YOU'LL NEVER BE TOO FAR AWAY
I'LL ALWAYS REMEMBER THE THINGS YOU HAD TO SAY
"SON, TREAT EVERYONE AS A BROTHER AND LOVE THEM FOR WHAT THEY ARE,
NEVER JUDGE THEM FOR THINGS THEY MIGHT DO OR SAY"
MY DEAREST GRANNY, YOU WERE A SPECIAL LADY, IN EVERY

SINGLE WAY

    MY LOVE FOR YOU WILL ALWAYS BE STRONG AND SURE ON EVEN   DARKEST DAYS

    MY LOVELY GRANNY, GOD BLESS YOU, AND AS WE SAY GOOD-BYE

    KNOW THIS: THE SEED OF LOVE YOU PLANTED IN ME WILL NEVER DIE

    MY ONLY GRANNY, YOU'LL ALWAYS BE MY SPECIAL LADY IN EVERY WAY

    MY LOVE FOR YOU WILL STAY STRONG FOREVER,

    NEVER TO FADE AWAY

I finished the song and closed my eyes for a moment. I didn't want to know if she had left me while I was singing. When I opened them I looked at her face, I put my hand on her chest and noticed she was still breathing. Then I saw it. The one thing that let me know she had heard my song; that she was still listening and had probably heard all of what we had said to her during the time she was in this coma. It was her lip. That wonderful upper lip of hers, that gave her emotions away each and every time. It was quivering like crazy. One huge tear escaped from her closed lids and rolled down her cheek.

"Oh, honey, I've loved you so, don't you ever forget it." Said George,, who had been sitting quietly on the other side of the bed, watching her and me through my whole performance.

I looked at George just then, to be sure he noticed her tear. He nodded and I knew that he had seen it. He bent over and kissed her and whispered to her for several minutes. I didn't want to listen to this last private, loving moment between them.

When George sat up, he said to me, "Best say your good-byes, son. The song was beautiful. I know she loved it."

I bent close to her again, and said once more, "I love you Granny." Then, I kissed her. As my lips parted hers, I felt her last breath. Her body was silent.

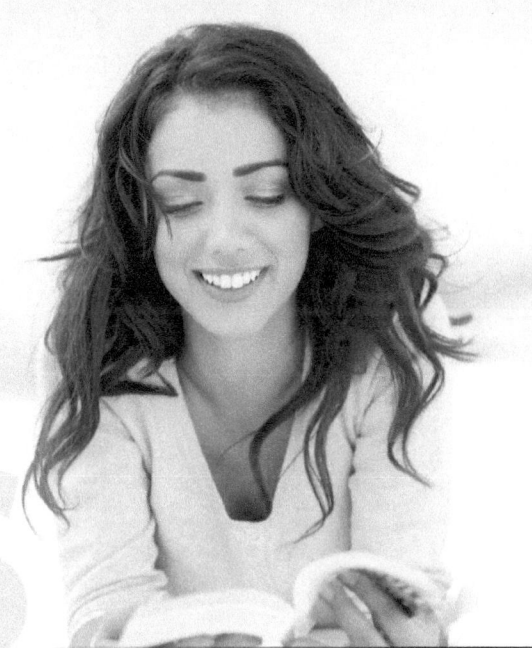

i want morebooks!

Buy your books fast and straightforward online - at one of world's fastest growing online book stores! Environmentally sound due to Print-on-Demand technologies.

Buy your books online at
www.get-morebooks.com

Kaufen Sie Ihre Bücher schnell und unkompliziert online – auf einer der am schnellsten wachsenden Buchhandelsplattformen weltweit! Dank Print-On-Demand umwelt- und ressourcenschonend produziert.

Bücher schneller online kaufen
www.morebooks.de

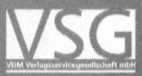

VDM Verlagsservicegesellschaft mbH
Heinrich-Böcking-Str. 6-8   Telefon: +49 681 3720 174   info@vdm-vsg.de
D - 66121 Saarbrücken   Telefax: +49 681 3720 1749   www.vdm-vsg.de

www.ingramcontent.com/pod-product-compliance
Lightning Source LLC
Chambersburg PA
CBHW020655220526
45464CB00001B/442